"...packs more of a strength-training punch than Pilates."

—*Fitness Magazine*

"Here is one equation that will keep you fit! ... In a one-hour [IM=X] workout, you can shape your legs, hips, abs, back, chest and arms... pro athletes, including members of the NY Mets use it..."

—*Physical Magazine*

"Where to do Pilates... IM=X."

—*The New York Times*

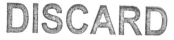

PILATES
FOR MEN

THE TOTAL SOLUTION FOR STRENGTH, FLEXIBILITY, AND POWER

PILATES
FOR MEN

ELYSE MCNERGNEY

CREATOR OF *im*=X PILATES

healthyliving**books**
NEW YORK · LONDON

CPL

A Healthy Living Book
Published by Hatherleigh Press
5-22 46th Avenue, Suite 200
Long Island City, NY 11101
www.hatherleighpress.com

Library of Congress Cataloging-in-Publication Data

McNergney, Elyse.
 Pilates for men : the total solution for strength, flexibility, and power
/ Elyse McNergney.
   p. cm.
 Includes bibliographical references and index.
 ISBN 1-57826-187-2 (alk. paper)
 1. Pilates method. 2. Physical fitness for men. I. Title.
 RA781.4.M38 2005
 613.7'1'081—dc22
                    2005002304

ISBN 1-57826-187-2

Disclaimer
Before beginning any exercise program, consult your physician. The author and publisher disclaim any liability, personal or professional, resulting from the application or misapplication of any of the information in this publication.

Pilates for Men is available for bulk purchase, special promotions, and premiums. For information on reselling and special purchase opportunities, call 1-800-528-2550 and ask for the Special Sales Manager.

Interior design by Deborah Miller
Cover design by Phil Mondestine
Photographs by Peter Field Peck

10 9 8 7 6 5 4 3 2 1
Printed in Canada

Acknowledgements

Special thanks to Lara Damadeo, Stella Hull-Lampkin, John Jay Wooldridge, Heather Craig, Chanda Fetter, Steve Smith, and all the other fabulous IM=X Pilates Instructors and Master Trainers who help improve the health of their many clients—and all of their many clients. I also want to thank all of the wonderful customers who have been so kind and dedicated to the IM=X programs. And a special thanks for the support and love from Rob and my dad.

Table of Contents

Introduction

Welcome to *Pilates for Men*, a core training workout for men! You probably have heard about Pilates from your friends' wives, who desire "ballet bodies," and thus have dismissed it. But, contrary to popular belief, Pilates was created by a man for men as well as for women. *Pilates for Men* combines free weights and stabilization with core training moves to fatigue you quicker than traditional Pilates. I created this home program with men in mind: fewer stretches, additional weight, no dancer moves, and a focus on trunk muscle endurance.

Pilates for Men uses the principles of IM=X Pilates, which has a proven track record for fast results and greater strength building. There are numerous testimonials from clients and certified personal trainers and instructors as to the intensity, uniqueness, and effectiveness of this intelligent approach to fitness.

My clients prefer IM=X because they know it is the most efficient total body workout that they can find. Orel Hershiser improved his fitness level during baseball season with it, Tiger Woods takes it, former Mets Strength Coach Barry Heyden selected it for his personal training business, and Bill Grant—former Mr. Universe—is an enthusiast. My very first franchisee—Steven J. Smith, owner of California Multisport—is a tri-athlete and proud owner of an IM=X Pilates Studio in northern California. These men know this is a powerful workout—one that cannot be found elsewhere.

It is also a safe workout, one that is easily adapted for use by men who suffer from injuries or just men who have been out of the gym for many years. Many of my clients have come to me with a back, hip, or shoulder pain. Often these ex-jocks are in their 40's or 50's and have been inactive for a period of several years. Weekend warriors, they continued to play their favorite sports but with no emphasis on conditioning their aging body. As a result, many were injured and then sometimes went through physical therapy but a post-rehabilitation workout routine was never prescribed. So these men returned to their old gym routines, only to become fearful of the resulting pain then they stopped exercising altogether. Pilates, along with the Alexander Technique, helped these men realign their joints (i.e. the spine, hips, shoulders), correct postural problems, and strengthen their weak links. If you suffer from joint pain or a similar injury, you can still use the sequences in this book—just eliminate the weights and focus on precision.

IM=X was deliberately designed to make Pilates more athletic and fitness oriented. It was in part designed for you—a man! For all of you who want rock-hard abs without the back pain, *Pilates for Men* is a solid program based on the science of core muscle recruitment and fatigue—endurance training for life. I have dedicated fourteen years to the development of this workout system, with the goal of providing something new and substantive in fitness that would address the universal aspects of aging, de-conditioning, and injury prevention. Through our many certified teachers and studios, tens of thousands of fitness participants have experienced the unique and powerful benefits of IM=X Pilates and here is what they say…

"IM=X Pilates is the best training and conditioning system that I have experienced. It has done more to relieve my chronic back problems than I could have imagined. My ability to participate in my favorite sports has been supported and enhanced and I plan on continuing indefinitely."

—*Sander Abend, M.D.*

"As a cyclist and triathlete, I'm looking to gain functional strength, improve flexibility, and prevent injury without spending hours in the gym. Integrating IM=X Pilates into my triathlon training program this past season helped me post career-best swim, bike, and run splits while remaining injury free."

—*Steven J. Smith*

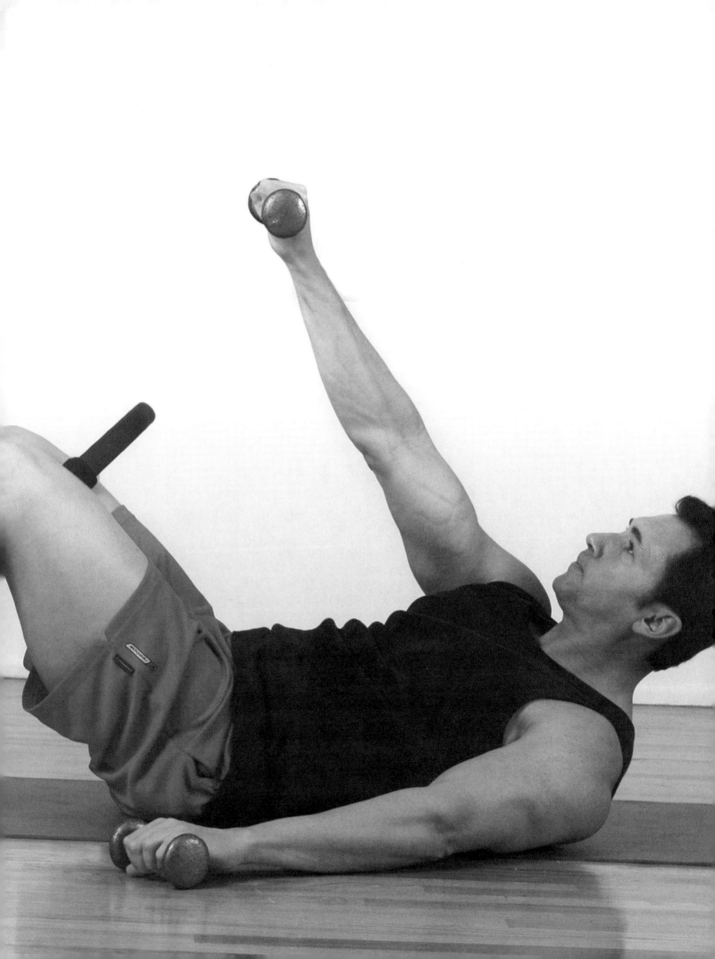

Why Pilates is Not Just for Women

Born in Germany in 1880, Joseph H. Pilates had been a frail child who suffered from asthma, rickets, and rheumatic fever. His illness convinced him to pursue fitness; he studied Eastern and Western forms of exercise in order to strengthen his body. During World War I, Joseph was placed in a "camp" with other German nationals where he taught wrestling and self-defense. In the camp, he began devising a system of original exercises to rehabilitate the many internees struck with wartime disease and physical injury. He invented a series of machines that operate against spring resistance rather than traditional weights. The main piece of equipment is called the "Reformer" and is still used, together with his original "mat work" or floor exercises.

The Pilates approach to conditioning and rehabilitation is highly effective for developing functional strength and endurance. Joseph's Reformer equipment utilized spring resistance because it conditions movement rather than single-muscle-building as occurs in traditional weight-training. For instance, the muscle coordination in a golf swing involves a series of motions/muscle patterns. The exercises on the Reformer mimic movement patterns seen in a variety of sports—the exercises improve spine strength in combination with limb motion, just as in a golf swing, a swimming stroke, or a skiing turn.

In 1925 Joseph decided to make the journey to America. En route he met his future wife, Clara, who became instrumental in helping him build his exercise program and business in New York City. Joseph and Clara opened a studio in Manhattan in a building that housed several dance groups. Joe Pilates became a fitness guru to the dance community. His powerful form of conditioning challenged the dancers' flexibility and coordination. Famous choreographers, including George Balanchine, Martha Graham, Ted Shawn, Ruth St. Denis, and Jerome Robbins, benefited from the Pilates system.

Joseph was truly an intuitive and creative exercise instructor who was indeed ahead of his time. While Americans were running and taking aerobics, dancers in New York City were taking Joseph Pilates's Reformer classes. Joe dedicated his life to developing exercise routines and equipment and remained fit up until his death in 1967 at 87 years of age. Now, over thirty years later, the faddish fitness press has turned Pilates into a household name and many teachers are continuing the tradition of Joseph Pilates.

In some ways my life has had parallels to Joseph Pilates'. I too have fought against illness. At the age of 20, while completing my undergraduate degree and a dance scholarship in Chicago, I became ill with a life-threatening bone marrow disease called aplastic anemia. I spent the next several years fighting for my life and using the power of movement to keep my heart strong. As a dancer, I was trained to perform fluid choreography that stretched the body and raised the heart rate. The combination of dance training and basic core training exercise helped me maintain some muscular and cardiovascular endurance (more strenuous training would have been dangerous in my condition because I was at risk for internal hemorraghing). These light workout routines saved me from becoming totally bedridden, allowing me to walk, climb some stairs, and stay hopeful. By maintaining a level of strength, I maximized my opportunities for survival—I also stimulated white and red blood cell production. With only a 30% chance of survival, I concentrated on building my ability to take in oxygen despite my desperately low proportion of red blood cells. It was life-affirming and powered my will to survive.

After undergoing chemotherapy, I was told that the treatment would either work or provide me with around 12 months to live. In 1989, despite the uncertainty and against doctor's orders, I moved to New York to pursue my dream of dance and movement. I had been an avid dancer since I was six, always relating to life through the joy of exercise. I figured that pursuing the Master's Degree in Dance at New York University would be the best way to affirm my life. My friends still tell me how horrible I looked in class, but, day by day, I built up strength through walking, praying and dancing.

It was during my recovery that I first took a Pilates class and discovered the core strength I had been missing. This inspired me to study at The Pilates Studio where Joe's pupil, Romana Kryzanowska, was training teachers. After completing the traditional Pilates certification offered at The Pilates Studio, I became fascinated with the science of movement efficiency. Energy efficiency was my main objective during my years with aplastic anemia. Because my recovery after the chemotherapy took about twelve months, leaving me with some permanent low-level anemia, I became intent on bringing energy efficiency into my dancing and jogging. This pursuit also led me to study the Alexander Technique, a body training technique designed by Frederick Milton Alexander.

Interestingly enough, F.M. Alexander and Joseph Pilates created their programs at around the same time in history. Totally different means to creating fluid motion and balance, they were to my mind equally powerful. These two methods surprised me in their ability to effect substantial change in my body—creating wellness and fitness. It also surprised me that neither method was being employed in physical rehabilitation and physical fitness. I was so excited about their ability to contribute to the fitness field and to cure back pain (I had many personal training clients who were completely cured of pain by the use of these two programs) that I decided to promote them.

Unfortunately my enthusiasm was met with scientific skepticism among the medical world. I was working at a physical therapy office and the doctors were wondering what the value of these strange techniques could be. This prompted me to dig into contemporary science to find the answers. I attended Columbia University to study Exercise Physiology with a focus on biomechanics and spine stabilization. It was within the walls of the library that I discovered a wealth of information on postural coordination, back stabilization, and muscle patterning for sports. Since my education in Pilates had not incorporated these scientific papers, I decided to create a certification course for teachers who were interested in the science of Pilates-style exercise—IM=X Pilates Certification.

IM=X stands for Integrated Movement eXercize. A cross-conditioning system that integrates resistance and cardiovascular training into Pilates moves, it is designed to increase flexibility, endurance, and muscle tone, while strengthening the spine and abdominal core. IM=X complements traditional weight-training, which isolates single muscles for development (a technique called hypertrophy), because it strengthens muscle synergies. Although traditional weight-training is important for maintaining muscle mass, muscle synergy training is important because it develops functional strength. When was the last time you isolated your *quadriceps* in a tennis match? How many times have you motivated your golf swing just from your *biceps*? Your abdominals and hip flexors work with your *quadriceps* for cycling; similarly, your upper back, shoulder and abdominals coordinate with your legs in a baseball game; and your rotational trunk muscles synergistically coordinate with your shoulders and arms to produce a perfect golf swing. In fact, you do not even stand without the help of your trunk stabilizers, so why would spend your workouts on your *deltoids* and *biceps* when you could train your whole torso and upper body simultaneously? Cosmetic muscle building accomplishes one goal, hypertrophy of single muscles, while Pilates-style workouts strengthen movements that improve your game.

Thank goodness muscles naturally work in tandem. Otherwise, we would be thinking "*erector spinae* contract, abdominals activate, left *quadriceps* engage…" just to take a step forward! But instead of laboring through conscious tedium, your brain is "wired" with a "muscle program" for twisting, curling, throwing, hitting, kicking and running. Your brain simplifies these activities for you but your muscle patterns may not be efficient.

An efficient way to hit a golf ball would include the IM=X principles to:

1) elongate your spine;
2) use a forced exhalation upon exertion to activate your core muscles;
3) power your arms in the swing from the trunk rotators, not from your neck,
4) focus on spine stabilization when you return to your starting position

The one efficient way to move is to recruit specific trunk muscles first before all other actions and to do so in a decompressed spinal alignment. Unfortunately, for most of us, this is not "natural" and does not occur during complicated sports moves. *Pilates for Men* will teach you how to do this.

The objective of this book is to provide a well-rounded home program that can be adapted in length and intensity for men of all fitness levels. I have also placed an emphasis on the fundamental exercises of IM=X because they address important aspects of de-conditioning and/or aging (i.e. joint weakness and decreased range of motion, shoulder and spine instability, spinal compression and loss of height)—all of which can be prevented with proper exercise. The workouts in this book are intended to be combined with regular cardiovascular exercise (i.e. walking, jogging, biking, cross-country skiing, kick-boxing, spinning, swimming, aerobics) and some weight-training.

As you read this book, keep in mind that the technique is what is important and the routine is simply choreography. In other words, although the exercises are designed in series to progress you through various joint ranges and target muscle groups, your ability to "feel" the detailed effort of the stabilization techniques is primary. These technique tips, which are introduced in Chapter 3, make up five fundamental principles for developing and maintaining a strong pelvis, trunk, and back. You are programming those muscles to work in the most efficient way, and you will want to build upon that programming to properly fatigue the muscles and get the most out of your workout. Commit to performing the exercises correctly and you will gain some serious core power and joint range of motion.

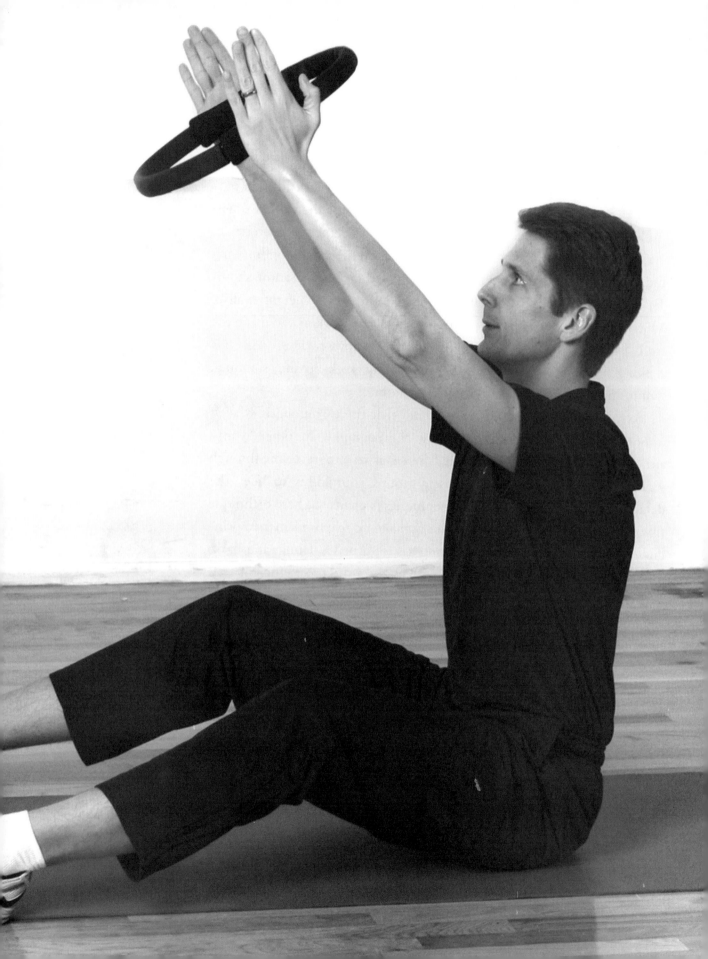

How to Use This Book

IM=X Pilates is a workout that combines series of movements—hence, Integrated Movement eXercize. In other words, you should follow the series as they are laid out in order to properly fatigue the muscles. If you selectively use the program by choosing single exercises from the routine, you will minimize your benefits. However, any exercise performed correctly is a good exercise, so you can still get results by performing shorter workouts if you don't feel ready for the full routine or are simply short on time.

The Series

The twelve series of movements in this book are designed to build upon each other with the initial series (the Foundational Series) designed to position the spine and teach the core muscles to activate in conjunction with the breath. In the Foundational Series, for instance, you will be working the deeper abdominal and pelvic muscles while in a lying position with your knees bent. Then you move on to Stretch Series 1, which loosens the hip and lower back muscles, so that you will be warmed up for Ab Series 2, which is performed in a lying position with your legs straight (which is tougher on your lower back).

You should always begin with the Foundational Series, which includes exercises to reinforce the five fundamental IM=X principles: Spinal Elongation, Forced Exhalation, Pelvic, Ribcage, and Spine Stabilization. (You'll learn more about the five principles in the next chapter.) From there, you can tailor your workout to be more or less intense depending upon your fitness level and what other types of workouts you plan to pair with your Pilates routine. Start with the Level 1 series, then add or move on to the Level 2 series, and then to the Level 3 and special (Lateral Moves and Spine Stabilization) series. At each level, you should start by performing the exercises without weights, then add weights when you feel comfortable with the sequence.

Each series targets a narrow set of muscles so that you can really focus upon building and strengthening those core muscles. Also, in each series, you stay in the same position to intensify the workout and make each sequence more efficient. In each workout, you will want to include at least one series that targets the abs, one that targets the back or spine, one that targets the hips or lateral moves, and one stretch series.

You will get the most out of your workout if you follow each series exactly. If you find any single exercise too difficult or painful, first try to modify it according to the instructions. If it's still a problem, then skip it and move on to the next exercise. However, please don't skip any of the fundamental exercises: Spinal Elongation, Forced Exhalation, Pelvic, Ribcage, and Spine Stabilization. These five fundamental principles will improve your skeletal alignment and program your core muscles to perform most efficiently and should be applied to every movement.

In order to retain muscle memory, you should do your *Pilates for Men* workout at least once a week; three times a week is optimal. Unlike traditional weight-training, in which you need to rest your muscles in between training days to allow them to recover, you could even do IM=X Pilates almost every day if you chose. Each workout in the program is designed to take just half an hour, but you can easily lengthen or shorten your routine by adding or skipping series according to the basic guidelines we've introduced here. See Appendix I for a 12-week basic fitness workout that you can use with any weight-training or cardio regimen.

How *Pilates for Men* Can Work with Your Traditional Fitness Program

This should not be your total fitness program. Pilates is for core strengthening and improving your range of motion at the joints. In order to maintain cardiovascular health, you will need to engage in heart-rate-training activities—i.e. run, play tennis, swim, bike, or walk. For more intense muscle-building, you should use weight-training equipment as typically offered at a gym. Pilates will provide you with the core muscle foundation and flexibility that you require to pursue all other sports activities and exercise programs.

Because IM=X Pilates emphasizes flexibility and extension, no warm-up, cool-down, or stretching routine is necessary to accompany these workouts. Instead, the workouts in this book can serve as a warm-up for your cardio or weight-training program. If you are preparing for a game, for instance, or are just planning on a kick-butt cardio workout, warm up with the Level 1 series to awaken your muscles and make your movements even more efficient. Similarly, you could use the Level 1 series after returning from a jog or bike ride to stretch and tone your muscles—thus avoiding stiffness or muscle imbalances.

Alternatively, if it's more convenient, you can choose to do your Pilates workouts on different days from your weight-training or cardio routines. Again, doing your *Pilates for Men* workout three days a week is optimal.

Take Your Time

In the beginning, perform the exercise routines at a slower pace. Once you are comfortable with the movement, then you may increase the speed. Again, though, remember that technique is primary so never move so quickly that you sacrifice proper form. That means making sure you apply the five fundamental principles and thinking about the internal muscle contractions you are performing.

The Foundational Series, which should be the first series of every workout, should take about 10 to 15 minutes to complete. Each of the other series should take between 5 to 8 minutes.

Equipment Needed

To start, you will need a pair of 3 lb, 4 lb, 5 lb, and/or 8 lb weights and a Pilates ring. The weights are used primarily to increase your core effort and will also strengthen your shoulders/arms as a secondary benefit. In other words, keep the weights light and focus on the total routine as well as the stabilization effort then increase to heavier weights. It is best if you can get two sets of free weights. On the long-lever exercises (with your arms stretched out—i.e. pec flies), use the lighter weights; on the short-lever exercises (with your elbows bent—i.e. bench press), use heavier weights. Do not go beyond the recommended weights, or you risk straining your neck.

If you are buying only one set of weights, choose based on the following:

- If you have rotator cuff or other shoulder issues, use 3 lb weights
- If you have limited range of motion (flexibility) in the shoulder joint, use 3 lb weights
- If you are sort of "out-of-shape," start with 3 lb weights
- If you have neck pain, use 3 lb weights

Bottom line, if you are just beginning the *Pilates for Men* program or have any kind of injury, use the lighter (3 or 4 lb) weights. After you have been using the program for several weeks, if you find that you are not fatigued after completing the Foundational Series and Ab Series Level 2, double-check to make sure you are recruiting your internal muscles properly and applying the five fundamental principles. If you are performing the exercises correctly and you are still not fatigued, then go up to the heavier (5 or 8 lb) weight. NEVER STRAIN YOUR NECK OR SHOULDERS IN ORDER TO COMPLETE THE WORKOUT.

Do Not Skip the Ring!

Sometimes when people buy our floorwork videos, they substitute pillows, balls or other objects in place of the ring. All I have to say is that they always wind up purchasing the ring later and then praising the workout. The program incorporates the ring not as a "bicep builder or thigh master" but rather for core stabilization. Men often take hold of the ring and compress it using their *biceps* and ask "Is this what this is for (ha ha)?" But then we have them lie on the floor with their legs extended, squeezing the ring, and using the weights to perform an ab curl. Let's just say their laughter at this time is no joke.

The ring, when placed between the inner thigh or ankle (depending on the exercise), is for core recruitment. Your *pelvic floor*, hip flexors, hip extensors (used in walking, biking, climbing—just about all leg movements), and lower abdominal region are all forced to work harder with the ring. Be careful not to "kill" the ring; over-squeezing creates the "thigh master" feeling instead of the manly "six pack."

My friend and former strength coach, Barry Heyden, used to call me during the Mets spring training and say "Send me some of those

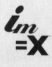

rings.... I am beginning their core training." The ring is an abdominal, back, and pelvic weapon not to be beaten by the *biceps* or inner thighs. When used properly, it facilitates maximum muscle fiber recruitment in the *illiopsoas*, *transversus abdominis*, *internal/external obliques*, *pelvic floor*, *quadratus lumborum*, *latissimus dorsi*, and lower *trapezius*, and even helps recruitment of the *erector spinae*—in other words, it strengthens your trunk muscles.

By focusing on using the ring for the internal recruitment of pelvic, hip, and abdominal muscles, you will be creating muscle patterns that will improve your back health and your golf, tennis, or racquetball game.

Choose a lightweight ring, preferably one with cushioned handles for an easy grip. Rings that are made of metal tend to be rather heavy and don't have as much "give" so they will not create the resistance you need. All rings are 14" or 15" in diameter.

The Mental Approach

The combination of:

1) applying the five fundamental principles introduced in the next chapter (Spinal Elongation, Forced Exhalation, Pelvic, Ribcage and Spine Stabilization)

2) the time frame in executing the routine (which gives you few water breaks) and

3) proper use of the equipment

will quickly define your muscles.

Your approach to this workout should be "yogi goes Rambo." In other words, you should challenge yourself but feel connected to the purpose of the exercises. If you do not take the time to connect to your *pelvic floor*, *transversus abdominis*, *internal obliques*, and *latissimus dorsi*, then you may strain your neck when you add weight. As you connect to the technique, you will increase the intensity and feel fatigued in the muscles targeted for each exercise. The good news is that by following the instructions in the book, you will understand how to challenge your core while improving your spinal alignment.

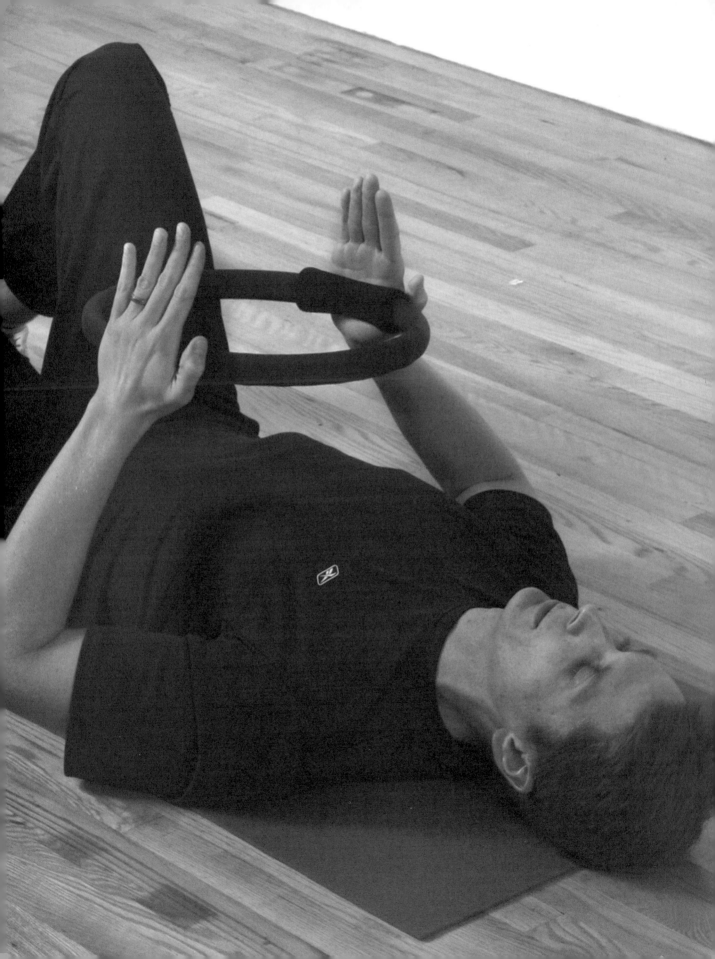

Getting the Most from Your Workout

In order to get the most out of your workouts, apply these universal IM=X principles to all of your exercise programs. These fundamental exercises will improve your skeletal alignment and condition the muscle firing patterns of your core to improve power and strength and decrease your risk of injury. Thankfully, the fundamental techniques are few. They are as follows:

1) **Spinal Elongation**. Used to lengthen the spine and hips during exercise

   In the long term, this prevents sports-related injuries that occur from muscle imbalances in the spine and hips. Also, this helps prevent poor posture that can occur with aging.

2) **Forced Exhalation Breathing**. Used to strengthen your *transversus abdominis*, *internal* and *external oblique* abdominal muscles, *pelvic floor*, and *diaphragm*. In the long term, this creates a strong trunk muscles that will work during exercise and protect your back from injury.

3) **Pelvic Stabilization**. Used to anchor the hips to produce strength in the hip and abdominal muscles; also creates stability for the lower back.

   In the long term, this prevents *pelvic floor* muscle from wasting, which is associated with aging and contributes to prostate problems or urinary incontinence.

4) **Ribcage Stabilization**. Used to prevent cervical compression and create stability in the upper back during arm and abdominal exercise.

   In the long term, this increases upper back stability during arm movements (i.e. weight lifting). Also, it provides effective muscle patterning for the protection of the cervical spine and for improved shoulder alignment.

5) **Spine Stabilization**. Combines the practice of pelvic and ribcage stabilization in order to anchor the spine during exercise.

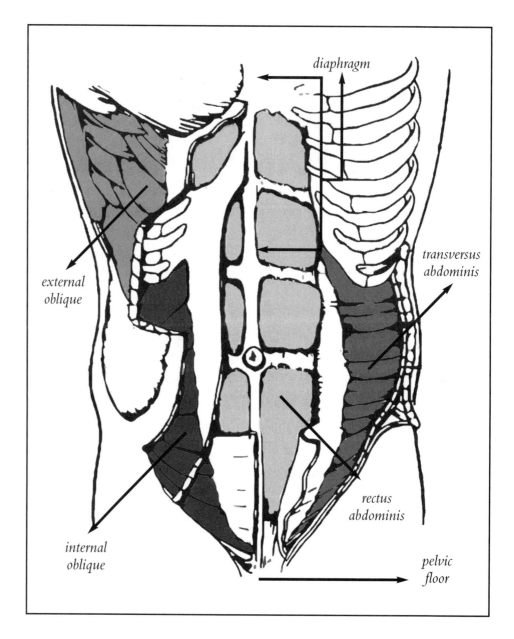

Core muscles

In the long term, this develops strength and endurance in all of your core muscles while improving your spinal alignment. Core muscles include the *transversus abdominis, internal oblique, external oblique, diaphragm, pelvic floor, iliopsoas, quadratus lumborum, latissimus dorsi,* and *erector spinae.*

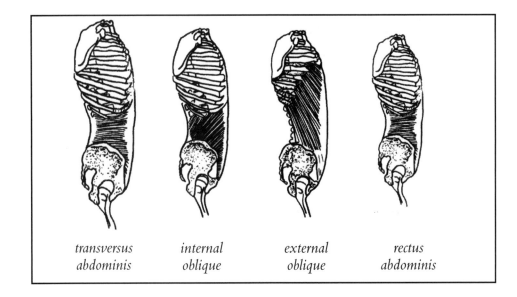

| transversus abdominis | internal oblique | external oblique | rectus abdominis |

As long as you grasp these principles and apply them to your workouts, you will improve your overall fitness level and develop a stronger center and back.

Spinal Elongation

Did you know that you are slightly shorter at the end of the day than after a good night's rest? And that research has measured a small degree of spinal shrinkage after weight lifting and running? The fact is we typically spend our days sitting in compressed positions with the spine at less than optimal length. We round forward over our computers, slump into one hip as we stand, and slouch when we sit. Over time this causes permanent damage. This exercise is designed to reverse these everyday stresses through the development of core muscle recruitment patterns that support length.

Throughout the book you'll be directed to elongate your spine by "reaching your arms and legs." Usually, you will be in a lying position, reaching your legs out of your hips and reaching your arms away from your legs to increase the length of your spine. By reaching your arms and legs, you are producing two opposing forces which decompress the vertebrae and hip joints, thus stretching them back into their optimal length. This lengthening action, especially when followed by a Ring stabilization exercise, helps build postural power. By creating more space between the spinal segments and at the hip socket (e.g. the *humerus*, or the *femur*), you will be fighting the aging process. Spinal elongation is the antidote to habitual shrinkage.

SPINAL ELONGATION

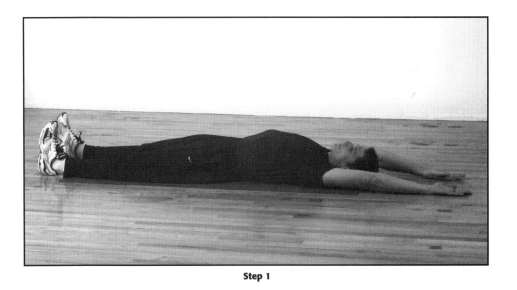

Step 1

Step 1. Lie on your back with your arms flat on the floor above your head and legs straight on the floor. Stretch your left arm and leg away from each other feeling the length of the hip and waist increase.

Step 2. Stretch your right arm and leg away from each other away, feeling the length of your right side increase.

Step 3. Stretch both arms and legs away from each other at the same time to lengthen the waist and hip joint.

BENEFIT:

Decompression of the spine and hips, improved posture, and prevention of spinal shrinkage which typically occurs with age and activities such as weight lifting, sitting, biking, and running.

GOAL:

Increase length in between the vertebrae and at the hip joints.

TARGET MUSCLES:

Transversus abdominis (deepest abdominal layer), *internal* and *external oblique,* (intermediate abdominal layers), *iliopsoas* (hip flexor), *quadratus lumborum* (lower back), and *erector spinae* (spine).

TECHNIQUE TIPS:

Notice the length in your spine and maintain it through the workout.

Getting the Most from Your Workout

Forced Exhalation Breathing

Forced exhalation breathing allows you to access the deepest abdominal layer, the *transversus abdominis*, and the intermediate abdominal layers, the *internal* and *external oblique* abdominals. If you are a "quiet breather," then this will be quite a change because the forced exhalation breath makes a little noise. But the difference it makes to your core training program is unmistakable.

The abdominal wall is comprised of four abdominal layers: *transversus abdominis*, *internal obliques*, *external obliques*, and *rectus abdominis*. As we grow older, our abdominal and pelvic muscles atrophy. A weak abdominal wall does not provide adequate support for the weight and bulk of the internal organs, which eventually push forward and expand the belly. Unfortunately, many traditional abdominal workouts do not reach the deeper support layers but rather focus on the more superficial abdominal muscle, the *rectus abdominis*. The forced exhalation breath recruits the three deepest layers, and sometimes all four.

Incorrect breathing will push the belly forward while forced exhalation breathing will pull all the muscles together internally. Thus, in order to maximize your abdominal tone, the forced exhalation breath must be consistently applied.

FORCED EXHALATION BREATHING

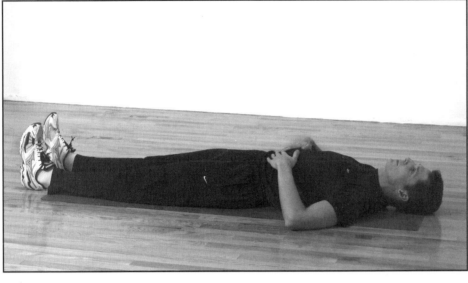

Step 1

Step 1. Lie on your back with your legs straight on the floor. Place your hands on your ribcage, and inhale.

Step 2. As you exhale, force the air out through pursed lips. As you blow the air out, contract the abdominal and *pelvic floor* muscles. This will not necessarily cause any visible movement since you are focusing on internal muscle contractions.

BENEFIT:

Training the core muscles to pre-contract before each exercise increases core muscle endurance and protects the back from the repetitive wear commonly associated with aging, de-conditioning, and sports activities.

GOAL:

Develop a breathing habit that maximizes core effort while reducing spinal compression.

TARGET MUSCLES:

Transversus abdominis (deepest abdominal layer), *internal* and *external oblique* (intermediate abdominal layers), *pelvic floor*, *quadratus lumborum* (lower back), and *diaphragm* (breathing muscle).

TECHNIQUE TIPS:

Use this type of breathing to strengthen these internal contractions while maintaining spinal length. With each inhale, breathe in deeply and lengthen through your back and torso. With each exhale, forcefully expel the air through pursed lips to contract your core.

Getting the
Most from
Your Workout

Stabilization Techniques

Stabilization means that one or more parts of your body are held completely still by an internal muscle contraction while other parts of your body move. There are three types of stabilization used in the foundation of IM=X Pilates—pelvic, ribcage and spine stabilization techniques.

The exercises look easy but when executed correctly, they enlist numerous muscles that are not usually engaged. For instance, it is rare that you would fully recruit your tranverse abdominis during an abdominal curl since this muscle contracts isometrically during curls but does not contribute to the lifting of your torso. Many of the most important core muscles support the internal organs but do not produce movement.

This workout strengthens both non-movement and movement-producing core muscles, including the *transversus abdominis, internal oblique, external oblique, diaphragm, pelvic floor, adductors, iliopsoas, quadratus lumborum, latissimus dorsi,* lower *trapezius,* and *erector spinae.* Your goal is not only to engage these muscles simultaneously, but to recruit as many fibers within each muscle by maximizing stabilization. The stabilization exercise is designed to teach you how to deepen your internal muscle contractions.

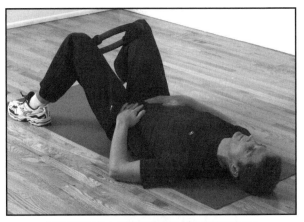

**PELVIC STABILIZATION
WITH RING**

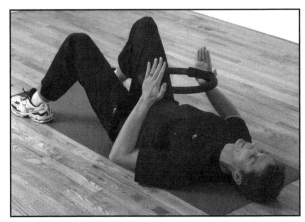

**RIBCAGE STABILIZATION
WITH RING**

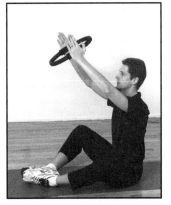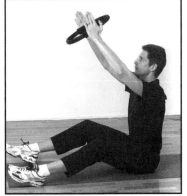

**SPINE STABILIZATION
WITH RING**

Pelvic Stabilization

Many people perform abdominal curls by hurling themselves forward rather than pre-activating the deep abdominal and pelvic layers. The spine actually receives an enormous amount of pressure if you perform crunches incorrectly. Research indicates that fast repetitive curls result in compression loads just under the National Institute of Occupational Safety and Hazards (NIOSH) guidelines for UPS workers!

In Pilates, you do not throw your elbows forward, pull on your head, nor buck your hips off the floor during abdominal curls. Instead, you initiate a curl with a forced exhalation and *pelvic floor* contraction while maintaining length in the lower back and further stabilizing with the *adductors* (inner thighs) and hip flexors by squeezing the ring. By anchoring the lower body with pelvic stabilization, you provide a stable fulcrum for conditioning trunk muscles and protect your lower back from unnecessary stress.

Pelvic floor strengthening is an integral aspect of the program—it simply makes sense to tone a muscle which otherwise weakens as a means of good prevention. Learning how to capture a good *pelvic floor* contraction requires conscious effort and practice. Since the *pelvic floor* is internal, there are no machines on the market to facilitate its strength. But since the *pelvic floor* and the deep abdominal layers act together, we are in luck! As you focus on recruiting your *transversus abdominis* with the forced exhalation breath, notice the activity in your *pelvic floor*—this is the essence of pelvic stabilization.

PELVIC STABILIZATION WITH RING

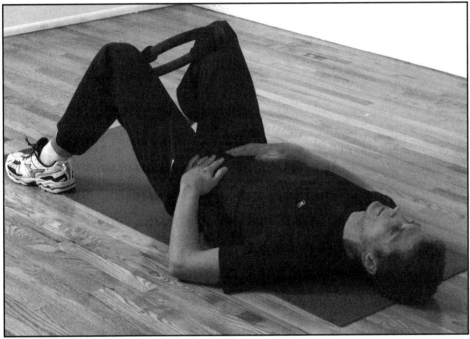

Step 2

Step 1. Lie on your back with your knees bent and feet flat on the floor. Place the ring between your thighs just below your knees. Lengthen your lower spine and maintain the natural curve in your spine (i.e., do not tuck your hips under).

Step 2. Reach your arms out to lengthen your spine. Then, place your hands at your hips so that you can "cue" your *pelvic floor* muscle.

Step 3. As you exhale forcefully, tighten your pelvic and lower abdominals. Note that this internal muscle recruitment may not produce any visible action—but you will feel the intensity of the effort.

BENEFIT:

Core muscle strength and healthy lower back alignment.

GOAL:

Lengthen the spine and contract abdominal and *pelvic floor* muscles at the same time to anchor the hips.

TARGET MUSCLES:

Transversus abdominis (deepest abdominal layer), *internal* and *external oblique* (intermediate abdominal layers), *diaphragm* (breathing muscle), *pelvic floor*, *quadratus lumborum* (lower back), *iliopsoas* (hip flexor) and *adductors* (inner thighs).

TECHNIQUE TIPS:

Deepen the contraction with each repetition—do not relax in between. If you are doing the exercise correctly, you will feel the contractions, the tightening within your hip and abdominal muscles, as you squeeze the ring. You should feel like you are working hard, that the intensity is building up with each repetition. However, keep your neck and buttock muscles relaxed.

Getting the Most from Your Workout

Ribcage Stabilization

Our cultural predisposition is to project our head forward. We lean forward as we talk on the phone, type at our computers, or even just listen attentively to each other. A "forward head" position is often accompanied by rounded shoulders. This damages the cervical and thoracic spine (upper and middle vertebrae of the spine). Making matters worse, our daily worries and anxieties are often deposited into our upper *trapezius* and neck extensor muscles. The fact is most of us respond to stress and demands by "tensing" and shortening the upper spine (not unlike a turtle pulling into its shell). Over time these habits can cause pain as muscles go into spasm and prolonged periods of spinal compression result in the shortening of the spine.

A shortened neck and hunched-up shoulders are the antithesis of ribcage stabilization. This upper body stabilization exercise is used to create a healthy position in the cervical and thoracic spine and shoulder girdle. By engaging the *transversus abdominis, internal oblique, external oblique, pelvic floor,* lower *trapezius* and *latissimus dorsi*, you will stabilize the ribcage for arm-strengthening exercises without tensing your upper shoulder.

The cue to "keep your shoulders wide and down" requires a mild contraction of the *latissimus dorsi* and lower *trapezius*. Practice widening your shoulders (rather than hunching them together) and lengthening your neck as you exhale—feel your *latissimus dorsi* and lower *trapezius* engage as you forcefully exhale. Repeat several times until you're clear where this additional pressing-down movement is generated—in the abdominal and back muscles, not your shoulders or neck. Make a kinesthetic memory of this muscle coordination and skeletal alignment.

*i*m
=X

RIBCAGE STABILIZATION WITH RING

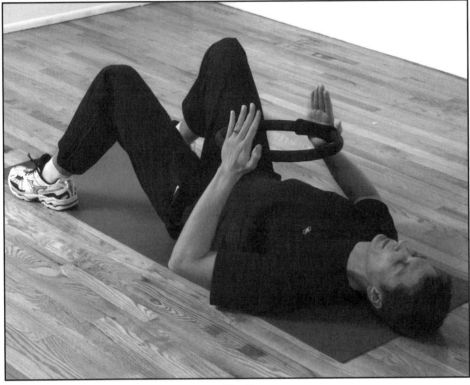

Step 2

Step 1. Lie on your back with your knees bent and feet flat on the floor. Hold the ring comfortably up in the air in front of your chest. Have your fingers long and relaxed, not gripping the ring. Direct your attention to the muscles around your ribcage.

Step 2. Inhale. Then, as you exhale forcefully, gently press against the ring. You should feel your abdominal, upper back, chest and shoulder muscles contract as you press.

BENEFIT:

Increased power in upper body movements (i.e. golf/tennis swing) and increased efficiency with upper body strength moves (i.e. lifting luggage, performing push-ups, throwing a punch).

GOAL:

Contract the *transversus abdominis, internal oblique, external oblique, diaphragm, latissimus dorsi,* lower *trapezius, erector spinae,* and other muscles of the ribcage while performing arm exercises. This aligns the cervical and thoracic spine for upper body strengthening (i.e. push-ups).

TARGET MUSCLES:

Transversus abdominis (deepest abdominal layer), *internal* and *external oblique* (intermediate abdominal layers), *diaphragm* (breathing muscle), *latissimus dorsi,* lower *trapezius* (upper back), *erector spinae* (spine), and other muscles of the shoulder and ribcage.

TECHNIQUE TIPS:

Your ribcage and shoulder girdle should be anchored, with all the surrounding muscles working except your neck and upper *trapezius.*

Getting the Most from Your Workout

Spine Stabilization

Sitting upright on the floor is a challenge for many of us. Chances are that when you sit down and hold the ring, your spine rounds, your shoulders rise up, and your head shifts forward. You may feel restricted by stiff leg muscles or a tight lower back.

To train your trunk muscles, you need to address your postural position. Sit on a chair or on the floor in a position that's comfortable, tilt slightly forward on your hip bone (the *ischium*, also called the sitting bone) and gently lengthen your spine. Be sure to relax your neck and shoulders while stretching up—imagine stacking your vertebrae one on top of each other. Reach and lengthen your torso out of your waist, creating more distance between your bottom rib and hips. Think of stretching slightly forward and up from your hips whenever you're in a seated position in order to extend your lumbar spine.

SPINE STABILIZATION WITH RING

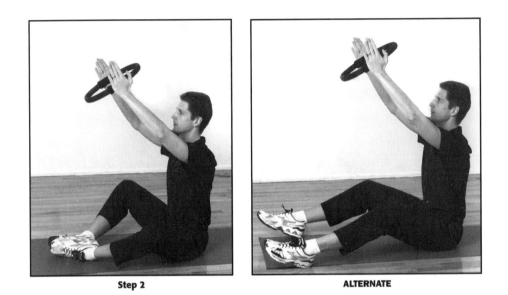

Step 2　　　　　　　　　　　**ALTERNATE**

Step 1. Sit on the floor with your legs in a diamond shape or shoulder width apart.

Step 2. Hold the ring lightly above and in front of your head. Keep your palms open and your fingers long and relaxed. Reach up, lengthening your spine.

Step 3. Inhale and use the forced exhalation to tighten your core muscles as you continue to reach up, pressing lightly against the ring. Repeat 4 times, concentrating on elongating the spine and deepening the core effort.

GOAL:
Lengthen and create isometric strength through all the core muscles.

TARGET MUSCLES:
Transversus abdominis (deepest abdominal layer), *diaphragm* (breathing muscle), *erector spinae* (spine), *pelvic floor, iliopsoas* (hip flexor), *quadratus lumborum* (lower back), *latissimus dorsi,* lower *trapezius* (upper back) and *multifidus* (back) muscles.

TECHNIQUE TIPS:
Do not lift your shoulders; rather, use your upper back muscles to lift upward. If it's easier, bend your knees slightly.

Getting the Most from Your Workout

Antidotes to the Top Ten Postural Mistakes

1) Moving the head forward (kind of like a pigeon does) when reaching upwards in a sitting of standing position: Practice Spine Stabilization with Ring.

2) Tucking your hips and rounding the lower back while sitting, standing, or performing an abdominal curl: Practice Pelvic Stabilization with Ring.

3) Raising your shoulders while lifting weights: Practice Ribcage Stabilization with Ring before using the weights.

4) Compressing into the hip joint during leg raises: Apply Spinal Elongation by reaching out of the hip joint prior to raising the leg.

5) Compressing the spine during abdominal curls: Apply Spinal Elongation by reaching back in between curls.

6) Slumping into one hip while standing or sitting: Practice Pelvic Stabilization with Ring in a chair.

7) Hyperextending your cervical spine when performing back strengthening exercises: Practice Spine Stabilization during back extension exercises.

8) Compressing the spine while stretching (for example, during a hamstring stretch): Practice Spine Stabilization during all stretch exercises.

9) Rounding the shoulders forward while sitting, standing, and weightlifting: Practice Ribcage Stabilization with Ring before using the weights.

10) Beginning an exercise without recruiting your abdominal muscles (core): Use the Forced Exhalation Breath to initiate each exercise.

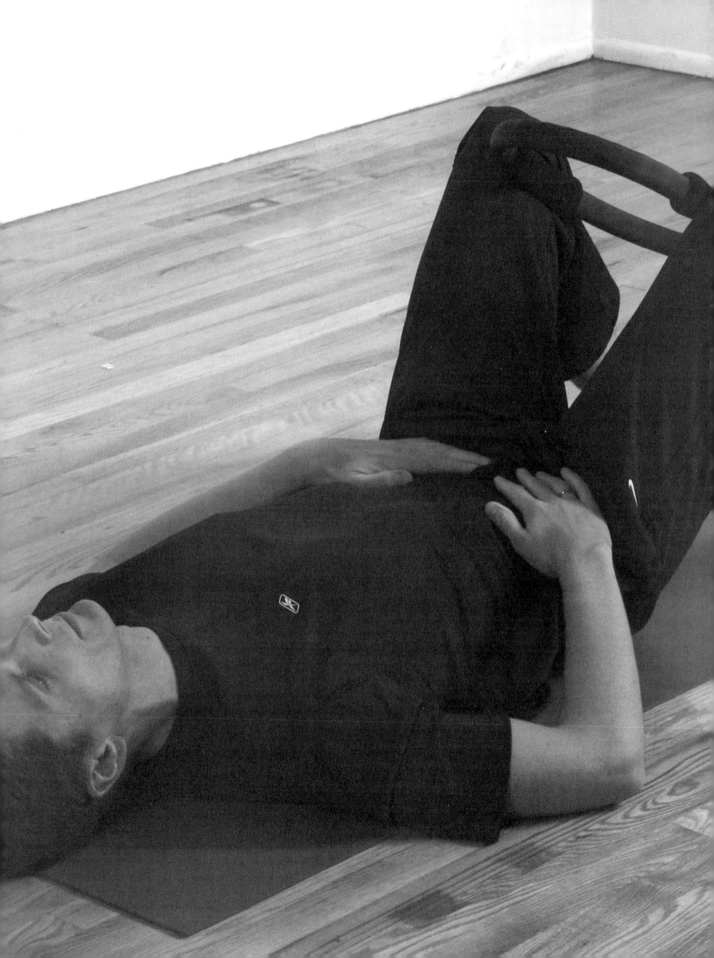

Chapter 4

Foundational Series
(Ab Series Level 1)

This Foundation Series uses the five fundamental principles to align your spine and hips to begin pelvic and abdominal core strengthening. The exercises are progressive so that you loosen the joints of the back before you start to develop internal muscle support. You will be working in a lying position with your knees bent. Start by performing all of the exercises without weights. Add weights only after you've mastered the technique.

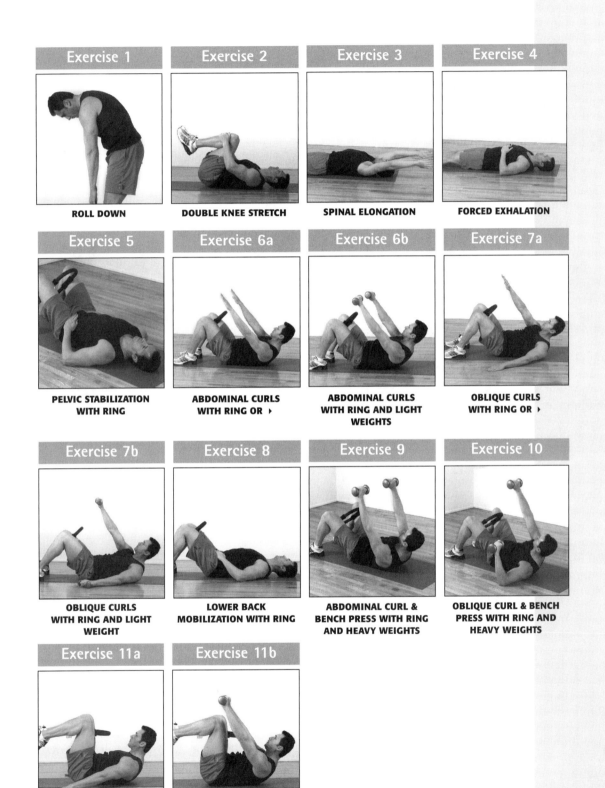

Exercise 1	Exercise 2	Exercise 3	Exercise 4
ROLL DOWN	**DOUBLE KNEE STRETCH**	**SPINAL ELONGATION**	**FORCED EXHALATION**

Exercise 5	Exercise 6a	Exercise 6b	Exercise 7a
PELVIC STABILIZATION WITH RING	**ABDOMINAL CURLS WITH RING OR ›**	**ABDOMINAL CURLS WITH RING AND LIGHT WEIGHTS**	**OBLIQUE CURLS WITH RING OR ›**

Exercise 7b	Exercise 8	Exercise 9	Exercise 10
OBLIQUE CURLS WITH RING AND LIGHT WEIGHT	**LOWER BACK MOBILIZATION WITH RING**	**ABDOMINAL CURL & BENCH PRESS WITH RING AND HEAVY WEIGHTS**	**OBLIQUE CURL & BENCH PRESS WITH RING AND HEAVY WEIGHTS**

Exercise 11a	Exercise 11b
REVERSE CURL WITH RING OR ›	**REVERSE CURL & BENCH PRESS WITH RING AND HEAVY WEIGHTS**

GOAL:

Warm up the spine and stretch the spinal and leg muscles. Decompress the spinal segments before abdominal training.

TARGET MUSCLES:

Erector spinae (spine), *quadratus lumborum* (lower back), *semispinalis thoracis*, and *multifidus* (back), plus *biceps femoris* (hamstrings) and *gastrocnemius* (calf) muscles.

TECHNIQUE TIPS:

Roll down through each part of the spine slowly so that you are using each joint in the back. Keep your knees slightly bent so that the soft tissue and muscles of the spine do not spasm. Use the forced exhalation breathing.

Exercise 1

ROLL DOWN

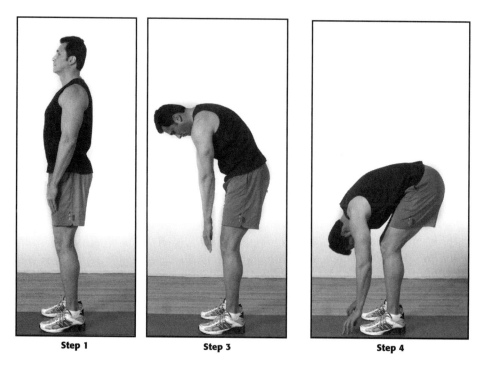

Step 1   Step 3   Step 4

Step 1. Stand with your feet hip width apart, knees slightly bent.

Step 2. Stretch your arms up in the air. Hold for a moment until you feel your back lengthen.

Step 3. Lower your arms to your side. With your knees slightly bent, bring your chin to your chest, roll your shoulders forward, and then continue to roll down through your spine, one vertebra at a time.

Step 4. Once you are all the way down, inhale and exhale as you reach towards the floor. Imagine that your spine is getting longer. Repeat until you feel that your neck, spine, and legs have been fully stretched.

Step 5. Exhale, tighten your abdominals, bend your knees, and roll up slowly. Again, as you roll up, imagine your spine lengthening and stretching up against gravity. Keep your weight slightly forward to keep your balance.

Step 6. Repeat if desired.

Exercise 2

DOUBLE KNEE STRETCH

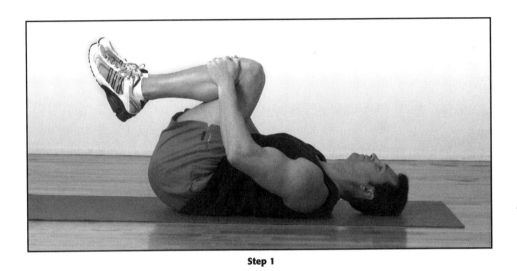

Step 1

Step 1. Lie on your back and pull your knees into your chest.

Step 2. Rock your legs back and forth gently to stretch your hip and lower back muscles.

GOAL:
Loosen the hip and back muscles before abdominal training.

TARGET MUSCLES:
Quadratus lumborum (lower back), *multifidus* (back), and *biceps femoris* (hamstrings) muscles.

TECHNIQUE TIPS:
Contract your lower abs as you stretch to protect the lower back.

Foundational Series
(Ab Series Level 1)

33

GOAL:

Increase length in between the vertebrae and at the hip joints.

TARGET MUSCLES:

Erector spinae (spine), *semispinalis thoracis, multifidus* (back), *latisimuss dorsi, quadratus lumborum* (lower back), *internal* and *external oblique* (intermediate abdominal layers), *rectus abdominis* (superficial abdominal), and *iliopsoas* (hip flexor) muscles.

TECHNIQUE TIPS:

Make sure that you feel the length through the hips and waist rather than lifting your shoulders to your ears.

im =X

34

SPINAL ELONGATION

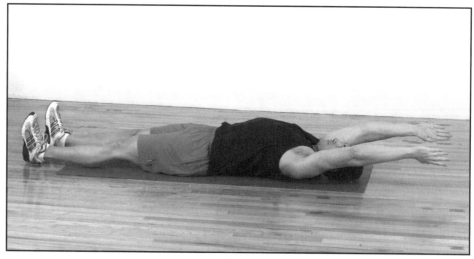

Step 1

Step 1. Lie on your back with your arms flat on the floor above your head and legs straight on the floor. Stretch your left arm and leg away from each other as far as possible.

Step 2. Stretch your right arm and leg away from each other as far as possible.

Step 3. Stretch both arms and legs away from each other at the same time to lengthen the hips and waist.

Exercise 4

FORCED EXHALATION

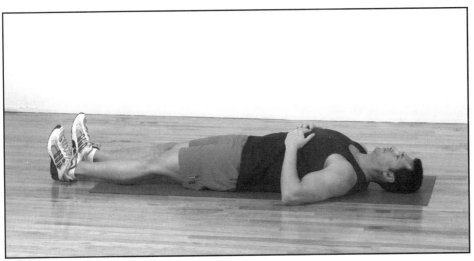

Step 1

Step 1. Lie on your back with your arms by your side and legs straight on the floor. Place your hands on your ribcage, and inhale.

Step 2. As you exhale, force the air out through pursed lips. You will feel your abs contract as you resist the outflow of air.

Step 3. As you blow the air out, contract the abdominal and *pelvic floor* muscles. Remember, this will not necessarily cause any visible movement since you are focusing on internal muscle contractions.

Step 4. Repeat for 3 or 4 breaths. Use the forced exhalation breath during your entire workout to deepen core muscle effort.

GOAL:

Develop a breathing habit that maximizes core effort while reducing spinal compression.

TARGET MUSCLES:

Transversus abdominis (deepest abdominal layer), *internal* and *external oblique*s (intermediate abdominal layers), *diaphragm* (breathing muscle), *quadratus lumborum* (lower back), and muscles of the ribcage.

TECHNIQUE TIPS:

If you are not making any noise as you force the air out, then you are not working hard enough.

Foundational Series
(Ab Series Level 1)

GOAL: Lengthen the spine and contract the abdominal and *pelvic floor* muscles at the same time to anchor the hips. Anchoring the hips provides a fulcrum for the torso to flex (curl) over. In other words, the pelvic contraction helps intensify abdominal training.

TARGET MUSCLES:

Transversus abdominis (deepest abdominal layer), *iliopsoas* (hip flexor), *pelvic floor*, and *adductors* (inner thighs).

TECHNIQUE TIPS:

Think of this as a pelvic and hip isometric contraction, rather than an inner thigh exercise. Do not round or flatten your lower back; instead, lengthen it. If you are doing the exercise correctly, you will feel you muscles tightening within your hips and abs, as you squeeze the ring. However, keep your neck and buttock muscles relaxed.

36

PELVIC STABILIZATION WITH RING

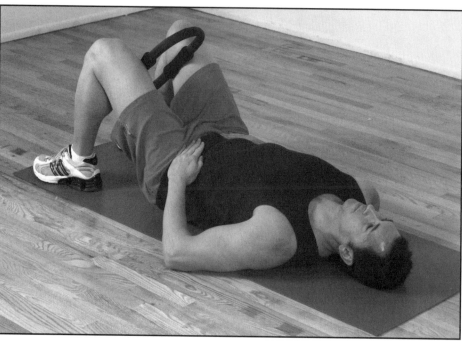

Step 2

Step 1. Lying on the floor, bend your knees with your feet flat on the floor, and place the ring between your knees. Lengthen your lower spine and maintain the natural curve in your spine (i.e., do not tuck your hips under).

Step 2. Reach your arms out to lengthen your spine. Then, place your hands at your hips so that you can "cue" your pelvic floor muscle.

Step 3. As you exhale forcefully, tighten your pelvic and lower abdominals. Again, you will not see much movement since you are focusing upon isometric contractions in the hip and pelvic muscles.

Step 4. Repeat 5 times, holding each repetition for at least 5 seconds. Deepen the contraction with each repetition. Do not relax your abdominal or pelvic muscles in between repetitions. The last time, hold the squeeze and continue on to exercise #6.

Exercise 6a

ABDOMINAL CURLS WITH RING

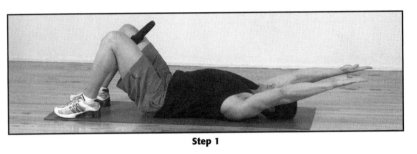

Step 1

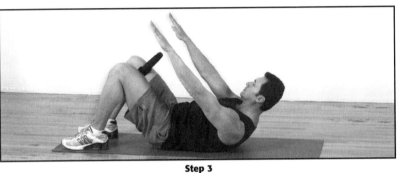

Step 3

Step 1. Still lying on your back and holding the pelvic stabilization from exercise #5 with the ring between your knees, reach your arms behind your head and stretch your spine. Take a moment to feel the stretch in your shoulder joint, and pull your shoulders down to the floor.

Step 2. As you exhale forcefully, squeeze the ring with your pelvic, hip, and lower abdominal muscles.

Step 3. Raise your arms, reach forward, and curl up until you feel your abdominal muscles working. This may only be a few inches, or you may come halfway to a sitting position. Your hands should come in front of your shoulders.

Step 4. Lower slowly back down to a lying position. Reach your arms behind your head and stretch your spine.

Step 5. Repeat 8 times.

OR

GOAL:
Strengthen the abdominal muscles while anchoring the hips.

TARGET MUSCLES:
Same as previous exercise plus the *internal* and *external obliques* (intermediate abdominal layers) and *rectus abdominis* (superficial abdominal layer).

TECHNIQUE TIPS:
Make sure to start with the breath to activate the *transversus abdominis* (deepest abdominal layer), *pelvic floor*, and *internal obliques*. Thus your abdominal curl is not being performed by your neck and shoulder muscles but rather by using the pelvic stabilization described in the previous exercise.

Foundational Series
(Ab Series Level 1)

37

GOAL:

Strengthen the core and lengthen the spine. The weights give additional resistance to your abs and help stretch your shoulders.

TARGET MUSCLES:

Transversus abdominis (deepest abdominal layer), *internal* and *external oblique* (intermediate abdominal layers), *rectus abdominis* (superficial abdominal layer), *iliopsoas* (hip flexor), *pelvic floor*, *latissimus dorsi* (upper back), *adductors* (inner thigh), *pectoralis* (chest), and other shoulder muscles.

TECHNIQUE TIPS:

Make sure that your feel your *latissimus dorsi* (upper back) working as you raise the weights. If your shoulders are up towards your ears, then you could hurt your neck. Use the breath to coordinate the movement.

ABDOMINAL CURLS WITH RING AND LIGHT WEIGHTS

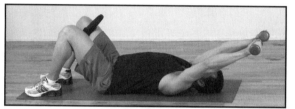

Step 1

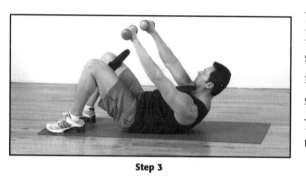

Step 3

Step 1. Still lying on your back and holding the pelvic stabilization from exercise #5 with the ring between your knees, take a weight in each hand, reach your arms behind your head, and stretch your spine. Take a moment to feel the stretch in your shoulder joint, and pull your shoulders down to the floor.

Step 2. As you exhale forcefully, squeeze the ring with your pelvic, hip, and lower abdominal muscles.

Step 3. Raise your arms with the weights in both hands, keeping your elbows straight. Reach forward, and curl up until you feel your abdominal muscles working. This may only be a few inches, or you may come halfway to a sitting position. Your hands should come in front of your shoulders (not down towards your hips).

Step 4. Lower yourself slowly back down to a lying position. Reach your arms behind your head and stretch your spine.

Step 5. Repeat 8 times.

Exercise 7a

OBLIQUE CURLS WITH RING

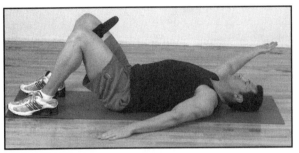

Step 1

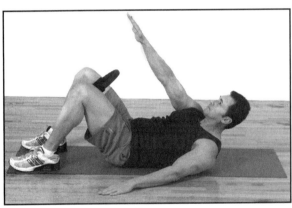

Step 3

Step 1. Still lying on your back and holding the pelvic stabilization from exercise #5 with the ring between your knees, place your right arm, palm up, on a high diagonal (about a 30-degree angle from your head) and your left arm, palm down, on a low diagonal (about a 30-degree angle from your left leg). Both arms should rest on the floor, or as close to it as you can comfortably come. Stretch your arms away from each other.

Step 2. As you exhale forcefully, engage your pelvic floor, lower abdominal, and inner thigh muscles to squeeze the ring.

Step 3. Reach your right arm across your body towards your left knee as you curl up until you feel your left oblique abdominals muscles working.

Step 4. Lower yourself slowly back down to a lying position. Stretch your arms away from each other and lengthen through your spine.

Step 5. Repeat 8 times, then switch sides to strengthen your right obliques.

OR

GOAL:
Strengthen the muscle synergy of the abdominal layers and hip area (useful in tennis, golf and other activities that require core power to rotate).

TARGET MUSCLES:
Same as the previous exercise but with a focus on stretching the shoulder muscles and strengthening the *internal* and *external obliques* (intermediate abdominal layers).

TECHNIQUE TIPS:
Do not move your hips. Instead, anchor your hips to the floor to control the curl. Also, remember to keep your neck relaxed.

Foundational Series
(Ab Series Level 1)

39

GOAL:

Increase the intensity of the oblique curl and stretch the shoulder joint. Maintaining range of motion at the shoulders is important for injury prevention.

TARGET MUSCLES:

Same as the previous exercise but with more focus on strengthening the *pectoralis* (chest) and *serratus anterior* (shoulder) muscles.

TECHNIQUE TIPS:

Remember the goal is to stretch the shoulder joint, not overload it with weight. A heavy weight could injure you, so be careful and focus on breath, core muscle recruitment, and shoulder stabilization.

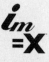

OBLIQUE CURLS WITH RING AND LIGHT WEIGHT

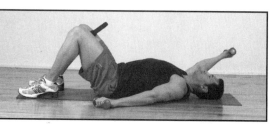
Step 1

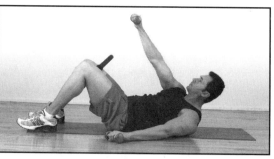
Step 3

Step 1. Still lying on your back and holding the pelvic stabilization from exercise #5 with the ring between your knees, place your right arm, palm up, on a high diagonal (about a 30-degree angle from your head) and your left arm, palm down, on a low diagonal (about a 30-degree angle from your left leg). Both arms should rest on the floor, or as close to it as you can comfortably come. Take a weight in each hand, and stretch your arms away on a diagonal.

Step 2. As you exhale forcefully, squeeze the ring.

Step 3. Reach your right arm, holding the weight, across your body towards your left knee as you curl up until you feel your ab muscles working. Use the weight in your left hand as a counterbalance.

Step 4. Lower yourself slowly back down to a lying position. Stretch your arms away from each other and lengthen through your spine.

Step 5. Repeat 8 times, then switch sides. (Note: You may want to begin with the side that you feel is non-dominant or weaker.)

Exercise 8

LOWER BACK MOBILIZATION WITH RING

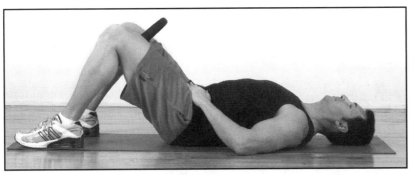

Step 1

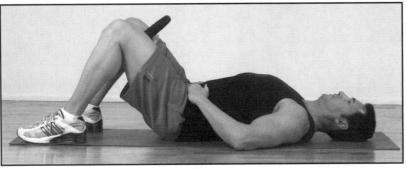

Step 2

GOAL:

Mobilize the lumbar spine and become familiar with proper placement. Research has indicated that lower back problems are more likely to occur if we lose touch with our spinal postures.

TARGET MUSCLES:

Erector spinae (spine), *quadratus lumborum* (lower back), *iliopsoas* (hip flexor), *transversus abdominis* (deepest abdominal layer) and *pelvic floor* muscles.

TECHNIQUE TIPS:

Go slow and use the exercise to lengthen your lower spine.

Step 1. Still lying on your back and holding the pelvic stabilization from exercise #5 with the ring between your knees, place your hands on your hips. Exhale and tuck your pelvis under so that your lower back is rounded. Simultaneously, tighten your hip and pelvic muscles.

Step 2. Inhale, lengthen the spine, and arch your lower back slightly. Keep the neck and shoulders relaxed.

Step 3. Repeat 4 times.

Foundational
Series
(Ab Series Level 1)

GOAL:

Strengthen the core with more intensity.

TARGET MUSCLES:

Transversus abdominis (deepest abdominal layer), *internal* and *external oblique* (intermediate abdominal layers), *rectus abdominis* (superficial abdominal layer), *iliopsoas* (hip flexor), *pelvic floor*, *latissimus dorsi* (upper back), *adductors* (inner thigh), *pectoralis* (chest), *serratus anterior* (shoulder), and *biceps* and *triceps* (arms).

TECHNIQUE TIPS:

Remember not to lead with the neck or shoulders. Instead, use the forced exhalation breath to initiate the movement. Again, if you are not making any exhalation noise, then you probably are not fully activating the core breathing muscles (abdominals, *pelvic floor*, *diaphragm*, upper back and ribcage muscles).

ABDOMINAL CURL & BENCH PRESS WITH RING AND HEAVY WEIGHTS

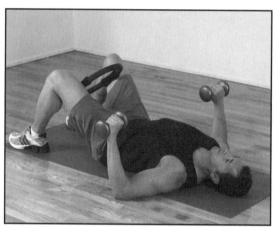

Step 1

Step 1. Still lying on your back and holding the pelvic stabilization from exercise #5 with the ring between your knees, take a weight in each hand. With your elbows out to the side (by your ribcage, not your ears) and your forearms perpendicular to the floor, hold your weights up on either side of your chest, palms facing forward.

Step 2. As you exhale forcefully, press the weights up to the ceiling.

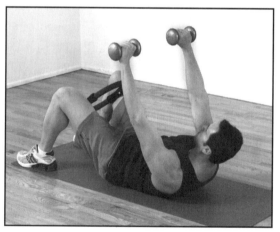

Step 3

Step 3. Holding the weights above your chest, exhale forcefully, squeeze the ring, and curl up until you feel your ab muscles working. Hold for a moment.

Step 4. Lower yourself slowly back to a lying position.

Step 5. Repeat 8 times.

Exercise 10

OBLIQUE CURL & BENCH PRESS WITH RING AND HEAVY WEIGHTS

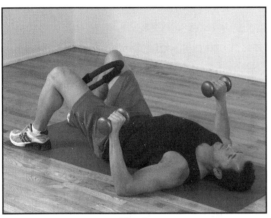

Step 1

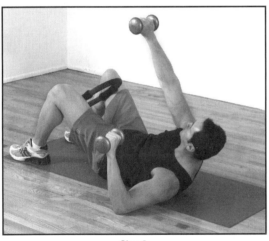

Step 2

Step 1. Still lying on your back and holding the pelvic stabilization from exercise #5 with the ring between your knees, take a weight in each hand. With your elbows out to the side (by your ribcage, not your ears) and your forearms perpendicular to the floor, hold your weights up on either side of your chest, palms facing forward.

Step 2. As you exhale forcefully, squeeze the ring and curl up extending your right arm. As you press the weight up your torso will rotate slightly to the left. Hold for a moment.

Step 3. Lower yourself slowly to a lying position returning the right elbow to the floor. Relax the neck and lengthen the spine momentarily before repeating Step 4. Repeat bench pressing the weight in the left arm 8 times, then switch sides.

GOAL:
Strengthen rotational muscles, which are important in tennis, golf, baseball, swimming, and volleyball.

TARGET MUSCLES:
Same as the previous exercise but with a focus on the *internal* and *external oblique* (intermediate abdominal layers) muscles.

TECHNIQUE TIPS:
Before performing the exercise, reach the weight up so that it is in front of the center of your chest. Make sure the weight is light enough to control the curl.

Foundational Series
(Ab Series Level 1)

GOAL:

Strengthen the hip flexors and lower abs. The main hip flexor is the *iliopsoas* (hip flexor). Research has indicated that a healthy lower back requires a flexible and strong *iliopsoas* (hip flexor).

TARGET MUSCLES:

Transversus abdominis (deepest abdominal layer), *internal* and *external oblique* (intermediate abdominal layers), rectus abdominis (superficial abdominal layer), *pelvic floor, iliopsoas* (hip flexor), and *adductors* (inner thighs).

TECHNIQUE TIPS:

Use the breath to control the movement as opposed to using momentum and speed. Force the air out and contract the abdominals to pull the knees in from the hip flexors.

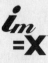

REVERSE CURL WITH RING

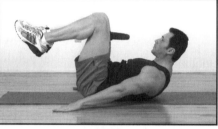

Step 3

Step 1. Still lying on your back and holding the pelvic stabilization from exercise #5 with the ring between your knees, set the weights aside. As you exhale forcefully, squeeze the ring, and curl up.

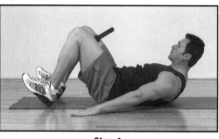

Step 4

Step 2. Place your arms, palms down, on a low diagonal (about a 30-degree angle from your legs). Press your hands into the floor to stabilize yourself while holding the curl.

Step 3. As you exhale forcefully, squeeze the ring and raise the knees in towards your chest. As you inhale, lower your feet to the ground. DO NOT LOWER FROM THE CURL. Simply raise and lower the knees while squeezing holding your curl and squeezing the ring.

Step 4. Repeat 8 times, then lower yourself slowly down to a lying position.

MODIFICATION:

If it's easier, you can place your hands behind your head to support your neck.

OR

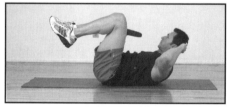

MODIFICATION

REVERSE CURL & BENCH PRESS
WITH RING AND HEAVY WEIGHTS

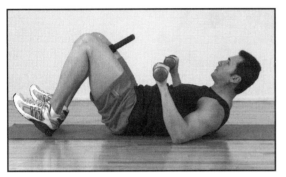

Step 1

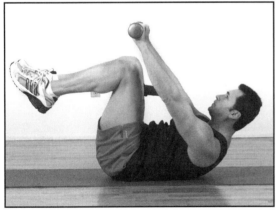

Step 2

Step 1. Still lying on your back and holding the pelvic stabilization from exercise #5 with the ring between your knees, take a weight in each hand. With your elbows out to the side and your forearms perpendicular to the floor, hold your weights up on either side of your chest, palms facing forward.

Step 2. As you exhale forcefully, squeeze the ring, curl up, and press the weights straight up to the ceiling while bringing your knees in toward your chest all at the same time.

Step 3. As you inhale, bring your elbows down and lower your feet to the ground but DO NOT LOWER FROM THE CURL.

Step 4. Repeat 8 times, then lower yourself slowly down to a lying position.

GOAL:
Strengthen all core muscles that are involved in trunk flexion. Intensify abdominal training by adding the ring and weights.

TARGET MUSCLES:
Same as the previous exercise plus the *latissimus dorsi* (upper back), *pectoralis* (chest) and *serratus anterior* (shoulder), *biceps* and *triceps* (arm) muscles.

TECHNIQUE TIPS:
Make sure that your arms fully extend in front of the chest in a parallel position; do not let them drift down or to the side.

Foundational Series
(Ab Series Level 1)

Chapter 5

Stretch Series Level 1

This sequence will loosen up tight hamstrings, hip, and lower back muscles. Remember: Do not compress your spine as your stretch your hamstrings and hip muscles!

Exercise 1	Exercise 2	Exercise 3	Exercise 4

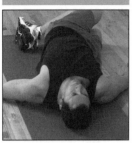

KNEE SIDE/EXTERNAL ROTATION/KNEE SIDE

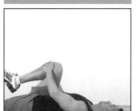

KNEE STRETCH

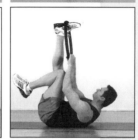

HAMSTRING STRETCH WITH RING

BENT LEG KNEE EXTENSION WITH RING

Exercise 5	Exercise 6

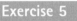
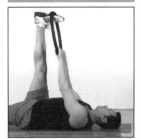

STRAIGHT LEG EXTENTSION WITH RING

LOWER BACK & HAMSTRING STRETCH WITH RING

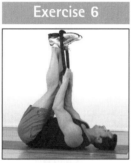

GOAL:

To stretch the lower spine and muscles of the hips

TARGET MUSCLES:

Erector spinae (spine), *multifidus* (back) and *quadratus lumborum* (lower back), *adductors* (inner thigh), and *gluteal* (butt) muscles.

TECHNIQUE TIPS:

Lengthen the waist as you stretch the lower spine. Make sure your lower abdominal muscles are working to support the stretch.

im=X

48

Exercise 1

KNEE SIDE/EXTERNAL ROTATION/KNEE SIDE

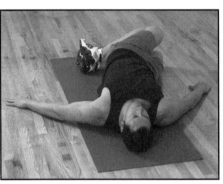
Step 2

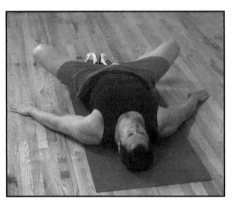
Step 3

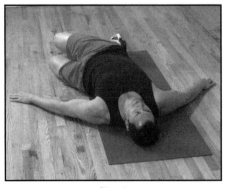
Step 4

Step 1. Lie on your back with your knees bent and your feet flat on the floor. With both arms on a low diagonal, press your palms down on the floor to stabilize your upper body.

Step 2. Bring your knees up to your chest, then lower them to the right side of your body to stretch your lower back. Keep your arms pressed down in order to achieve the shoulder stretch and stabilize the upper back. You can either keep your head neutral or look toward the left.

Step 3. Open the left leg so that your left knee points toward the left side of your body. Hold for a moment to stretch your inner thigh/groin muscles.

Step 4. Close the right leg over to the left so that both knees point toward the left side of your body to stretch your lower back on the other side.

Step 5. Repeat once in each direction.

Exercise 2

KNEE STRETCH

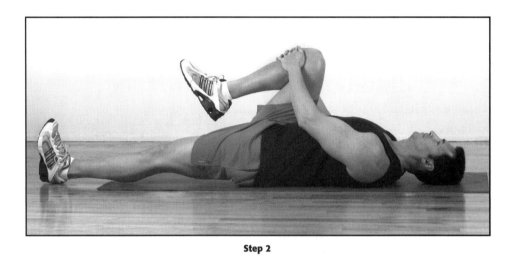

Step 2

Step 1. Lie on your back with your arms flat on the floor above your head and legs straight on the floor. Lengthen your spine by reaching your fingers and toes away from each other as far as possible.

Step 2. As you exhale, pull your right knee into your chest, using your hands to hold the stretch while keeping the left leg extended and pressed down into the floor.

Step 3. Inhale, release the stretch, and return to your starting position.

Step 4. Repeat 3 times, then change sides.

GOAL:

Stretch the hip and lower back region.

TARGET MUSCLES:

Erector spinae (spine), *multifidus* (back) and *quadratus lumborum* (lower back), *iliopsoas* (hip flexor) and *biceps femoris* (hamstrings).

TECHNIQUE TIPS:

Try not to flatten your lower back by rotating the hips under; instead, maintain the length in your spine. When you isolate the stretch, you accomplish your flexibility goals quicker.

Stretch Series
Level 1

GOAL:

Increase the flexibility of the hamstrings, hips, and lower back.

TARGET MUSCLES:

Erector spinae (spine), *multifidus* (back), *quadratus lumborum* (lower back), *biceps femoris* (hamstring), *gastrocnemius* and *soleus* (calf) muscles.

TECHNIQUE TIPS:

Try not to flatten your lower back by tucking the hips under. Instead, maintain the length in your lumbar spine to isolate the stretch and keep your shoulders down.

NOTE: The following sequence of stretches should be completed with one leg before changing to the other side. Starting with your right side perform exercises and then repeat on the left side before proceeding to exercise #6. The goals, #3 through #5 target muscles, and technique tips are the same for exercises #3 through #6.

Exercise 3

HAMSTRING STRETCH WITH RING

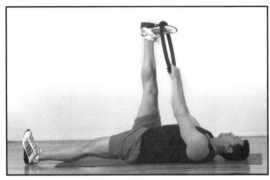

Step 1

Step 1. Still lying on your back with your left leg straight on the floor, place your right foot into the ring, tighten your abdominals, and extend your leg to the ceiling.

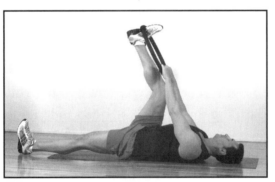

Step 2

Step 2. Inhale and bend your right knee, pulling your thigh a little closer towards your chest.

Step 3. Repeat 3 times and hold to go on to exercise #4.

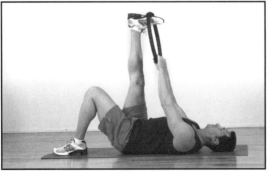

MODIFICATION

MODIFICATION:

If it's easier, you can bend your left leg.

im
=X

Exercise 4

BENT LEG KNEE EXTENSION WITH RING

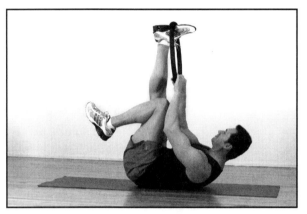

Step 1

Step 1. Holding the hamstring stretch on your right side, exhale forcefully, bend your left knee in toward your chest, tighten your abdominals, and curl up until you feel your abdominals working.

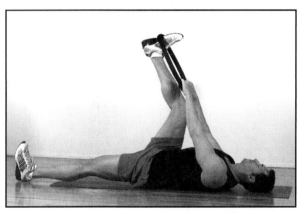

Step 2

Step 2. As you inhale, lower yourself back down from the curl and straighten your left leg, pressing into the floor.

Step 3. Repeat 3 times and hold to go on to exercise #5.

Stretch Series
Level 1

51

STRAIGHT LEG EXTENSION WITH RING

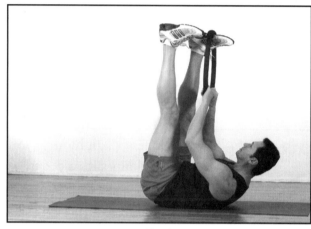

Step 1

This is the same exercise as #4 but with your legs straight.

Step 1. Still holding the hamstring stretch on your right side, exhale forcefully, bring your left leg toward your chest, tighten your abdominals, and curl up until you feel your abdominals working. Keep your left leg as straight as possible.

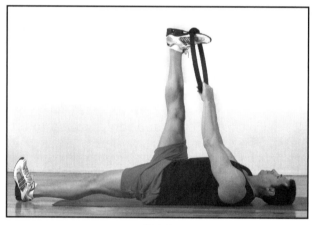

Step 2

Step 2. As you inhale, lower yourself back down from the curl and lower your left leg, pressing it into the floor.

Step 3. Repeat 3 times.

Step 4. Repeat exercises #3 through #5 on the left side.

LOWER BACK & HAMSTRING STRETCH WITH RING

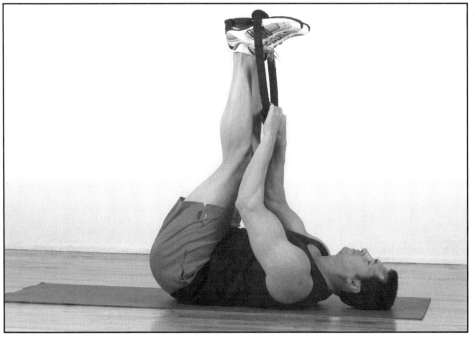

Step 2

Step 1. Lie on your back and place both feet in the ring, extending your legs toward the ceiling.

Step 2. Exhale and pull your legs in toward your chest, bending your knees as necessary, for a lower back and hamstring stretch.

Step 3. Repeat 3 times.

Stretch Series
Level 1

Chapter 6

Ab Series
Level 2

Now that you know the basics, your core conditioning program will intensify. As the levels progress, concentrate on the principles and think of how well you are executing an exercise, not how many times. You may not be able to reach as far or curl up as high as you see in the photos but that is okay. A small range of motion or fewer repetitions is far superior when done with proper breathing and stabilization. And, as always, if your neck or back hurts, stop immediately.

Exercise 1	Exercise 2a	Exercise 2b	Exercise 3a
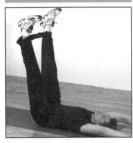	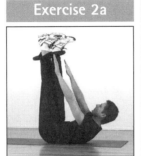	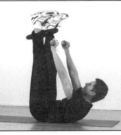	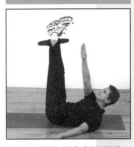
CORE RECRUITMENT WITH RING	**EXTENDED LEG ABDOMINAL CURLS WITH RING OR ▸**	**EXTENDED LEG ABDOMINAL CURLS WITH RING AND LIGHT WEIGHTS**	**EXTENDED LEG OBLIQUE CURLS WITH RING OR ▸**

Exercise 3b	Exercise 4	Exercise 5	Exercise 6
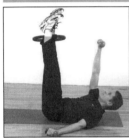	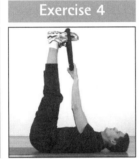	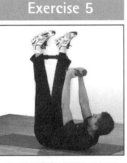	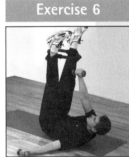
EXTENDED LEG OBLIQUE CURLS WITH RING AND LIGHT WEIGHTS	**LOWER BACK & HAMSTRING STRETCH WITH RING**	**ABDOMINAL CURL & PEC FLIES WITH RING AND LIGHT WEIGHTS**	**OBLIQUE CURL & PEC FLIES WTIH RING AND LIGHT WEIGHTS**

Exercise 7	Exercise 8
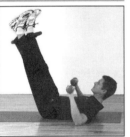	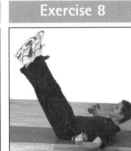
EXTENDED LEG REVERSE CURL & BENCH PRESS WITH RING AND HEAVY WEIGHTS	**EXTENDED LEG REVERSE CURL & PEC FLIES WITH RING AND HEAVY WEIGHTS**

GOAL:

Increase flexibility of the hamstrings and lower back.

TARGET MUSCLES:

Transversus abdominis (deepest abdominal layer), *diaphragm* (breathing muscle), *multifidus* (back), *quadratus lumborum* (lower back), *iliopsoas* (hip flexor), *biceps femoris* (hamstrings), *pelvic floor,* and *adductors* (inner thighs).

TECHNIQUE TIPS:

Keep your shoulders down and your spine long.

CORE RECRUITMENT WITH RING

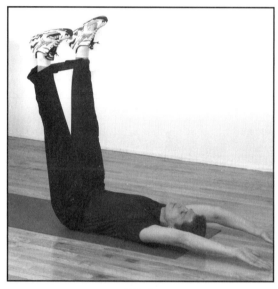

Step 1

Step 1. Lie on your back bring your knees in toward your chest, place the ring between your ankles, and extend your legs straight up to the ceiling, externally rotating your thighs from your hip, not your knees. Reach your arms overhead.

Step 2. Exhale forcefully and squeeze the ring, reaching arms away from your legs in order to lengthen the spine.

Step 3. Hold for 4 deep exhalations, then go directly onto exercise #2.

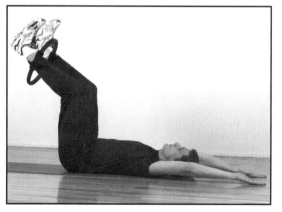

MODIFICATION

MODIFICATION: If you feel any discomfort in the lower back, bend your knees slightly.

EXTENDED LEG ABDOMINAL CURLS WITH RING

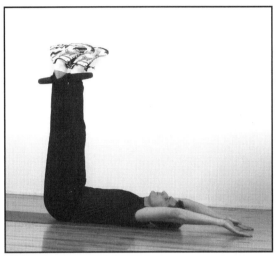

Step 1

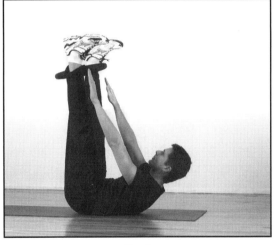

Step 2

Step 1. Still lying on your back with the ring between your ankles and legs straight up in the air, stretch your arms overhead.

Step 2. Exhale forcefully, squeeze the ring, and curl up.

Step 3. Inhale, reach back to the starting position, keeping your legs straight up.

Step 4. Repeat 8 times.

OR

GOAL:

Strengthen the *transversus abdominis* (deepest abdominal layer), *internal* and *external* obliques (intermediate abdominal layers), *rectus abdominis* (superficial abdominal layer), while increasing flexibility in the legs.

TARGET MUSCLES:

Same as the previous exercise but with a focus on *transversus abdominis* (deepest abdominal layer), *internal* and *external* obliques (intermediate abdominal layers), *rectus abdominis* (superficial abdominal layer).

TECHNIQUE TIPS:

Use the forced exhalation to contract the muscles of the hips as you squeeze the ring. If it's easier, place your hands behind your head

Ab Series
Level 2

GOAL:

Stretch the shoulder joint while strengthening the core.

TARGET MUSCLES:

Same as the previous exercise plus *deltoids* (shoulder), lower *trapezius* (upper back) and *pectoralis* (chest) muscles.

TECHNIQUE TIPS:

Keep your shoulders down and your neck muscles relaxed. Use your upper back muscles to lift the weights. And use the forced exhalation breath to contract your abdominals before you raise your arms up.

EXTENDED LEG ABDOMINAL CURLS WITH RING AND LIGHT WEIGHTS

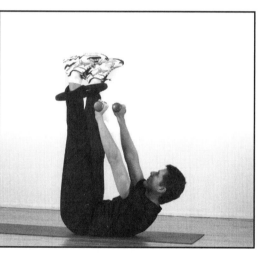

Step 1

Step 2

Step 1. Still lying on your back with the ring between your ankles and legs straight up in the air, take a weight in each hand. Your arms should be flat on the floor above your head, palms facing up.

Step 2. Exhale forcefully, squeeze the ring, and curl up with your arms straight until your head and shoulders come off the floor. Your arms should stop in front of your chest.

Step 3. As you inhale, reach slowly back to your starting position, making sure to keep your legs straight up in the air. Take a moment to feel the stretch in your shoulder joint.

Step 4. Repeat 8 times.

im
=X

EXTENDED LEG OBLIQUE CURLS WITH RING

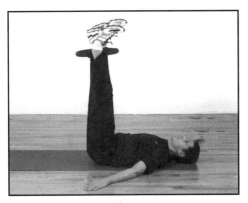

Step 1

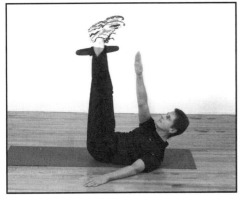

Step 2

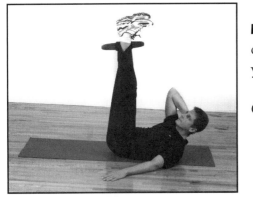

MODIFICATION

Step 1. Still lying on your back with the ring between your ankles and legs straight up in the air, place your right hand, palm up, on a high diagonal and your left hand, palm down, on a low diagonal.

Step 2. Exhale forcefully, squeeze the ring, and reach your right arm across your body toward your left knee as you curl up just until your neck and shoulders come off the floor.

Step 3. As you inhale, lower yourself slowly back to your starting position, making sure to keep your legs straight up.

Step 4. Repeat 8 times, then switch sides.

MODIFICATION: If it helps, you can place your right hand behind your head to support your neck.

OR

GOAL:

Strengthen the muscle synergy of the abdominal layers and hip area, which will be useful in tennis, golf, and other activities that require core power to rotate.

TARGET MUSCLES:

Transversus abdominis (deepest abdominal layer), *diaphragm* (breathing muscle), *iliopsoas* (hip flexor), *biceps femoris* (hamstrings), *pelvic floor* and *adductors* (inner thighs).

TECHNIQUE TIPS:

Do not move your hips. Instead, anchor your hips to control the curl.

Ab Series
Level 2

GOAL:

Increase the intensity of the oblique curl and stretch the shoulder joint. Maintaining range of motion at the shoulders is important for injury prevention.

TARGET MUSCLES:

Same as the previous exercise plus *latissimus dorsi* (upper back), lower *trapezius* (upper back), *pectoralis* (chest), and *deltoids* (shoulder) muscles.

TECHNIQUE TIPS:

Remember that the goal is to stretch the shoulder joint, not overload it with weight. A heavy weight could injure you, so be careful and focus on core muscle recruitment and shoulder stabilization.

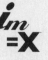

EXTENDED LEG OBLIQUE CURLS WITH RING AND LIGHT WEIGHTS

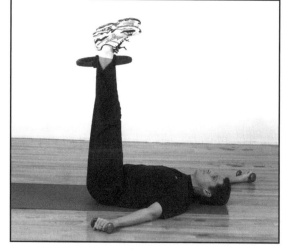

Step 1

Step 1. Still lying on your back with the ring between your ankles and legs straight up in the air, take a weight in each hand. Place your right hand, palm up, on a high diagonal and your left hand, palm down, on a low diagonal.

Step 2. Exhale forcefully, squeeze the ring, reach your right arm across your body toward your left knee, and curl up.

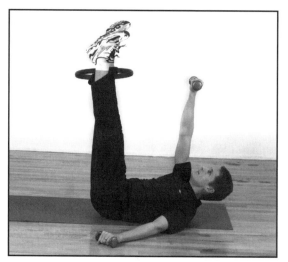

Step 2

Step 3. As you inhale, lower yourself slowly back to your starting position, making sure to keep your legs straight up.

Step 4. Repeat 8 times, then switch sides.

Exercise 4

LOWER BACK & HAMSTRING STRETCH WITH RING

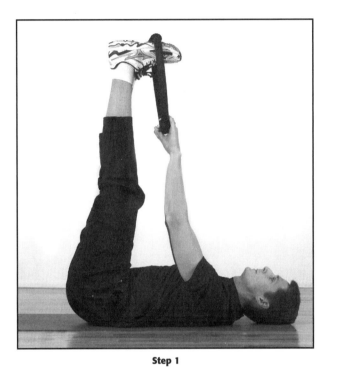

Step 1

Step 1. Lie on your back and place both feet in the ring, extending your legs toward the ceiling.

Step 2. Exhale and pull your legs in toward your chest, keeping them as straight as possible. You will feel the stretch in your lower back and legs.

Step 3. Repeat 3 times.

GOAL:

Increase flexibility in the legs, hips, and lower spine.

TARGET MUSCLES:

Erector spinae (spine), *multifidus* (back) and *quadratus lumborum* (lower back), *biceps femoris* (hamstring), *gastrocnemius* and *soleus* (calf) muscles.

TECHNIQUE TIPS:

Try not to flatten your lower back by tucking the hips under. Instead, maintain the length in your lumbar spine to isolate the stretch and keep your shoulders down.

Ab Series
Level 2

GOAL:

Strengthen your core and shoulder muscles.

TARGET MUSCLES:

Transversus abdominis (deepest abdominal layer), *internal* and *external* obliques (intermediate abdominal layers), *rectus abdominis* (superficial abdominal layer), *diaphragm* (breathing muscle), *iliopsoas* (hip flexor), *biceps femoris* (hamstrings), *pelvic floor* and *adductors* (inner thighs), *latissums dorsi*, lower *trapezius* (upper back), and *pectoralis* (chest) muscles.

TECHNIQUE TIPS:

Keep your shoulders down and ribcage stabilized.

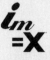

ABDOMINAL CURL & PEC FLIES WITH RING AND LIGHT WEIGHTS

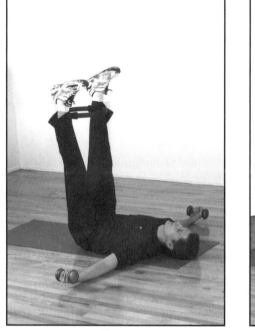

Step 1

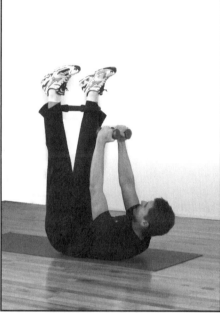

Step 2

Step 1. Still lying on your back, place the ring between your ankles and extend your legs straight up in the air. Hold a weight in each hand, palms facing each other, with your arms out to the side and elbows slightly bent.

Step 2. Exhale forcefully, squeeze the ring, and arc your arms up until they are directly over your chest, keeping your elbows rounded, as if you were hugging a big tree. At the same time, curl up just until your head and shoulders come off the floor.

Step 3. As you inhale, lower yourself slowly back to your starting position, making sure to keep your legs straight up in the air.

Step 4. Repeat 8 times.

OBLIQUE CURL & PEC FLIES
WITH RING AND LIGHT WEIGHTS

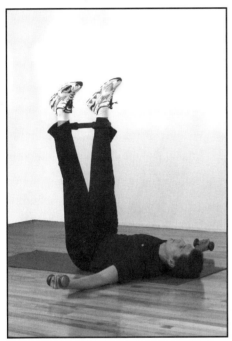

Step 1

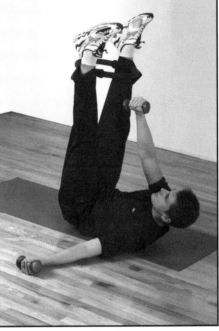

Step 2

GOAL:
Maintain pelvic stabilization while improving rotational strength.

TARGET MUSCLES:
Same as the previous exercise but with a focus on the *oblique* abdominals.

TECHNIQUE TIPS:
If your abdominal and hip muscles are extremely sore from the previous exercise, rest for a few minutes before performing this exercise.

Step 1. Still lying on your back, place the ring between your ankles and extend your legs straight up in the air. Hold a weight in each hand, palms facing each other, with your arms out to the side and elbows slightly bent.

Step 2. Exhale forcefully, squeeze the ring, and arc your right arm up in a one-arm hug. At the same time, curl up toward your left knee until you feel your left oblique abdominals working.

Step 3. As you inhale, lower yourself slowly back to your starting position, making sure to keep your legs straight up.

Step 4. Repeat 8 times, then switch sides.

Ab Series
Level 2

GOAL:

Strengthen the abdominal wall, hip flexors, and thighs.

TARGET MUSCLES:

Transversus abdominis (deepest abdominal layer), *internal* and *external* obliques (intermediate abdominal layers), *rectus abdominis* (superficial abdominal layer), *iliopsoas* (hip flexor), adductor (inner thigh *pelvic floor*, *pectoralis* (chest), *deltoids* (shoulder), *biceps* and *triceps* (arms).

TECHNIQUE TIPS:

If you feel any discomfort in your lower back as you perform the exercise, stop and pull your knees into your chest. Concentrate on using your abdominal muscles to move your legs, instead of lifting your pelvis.

64

EXTENDED LEG REVERSE CURL & BENCH PRESS WITH RING AND HEAVY WEIGHTS

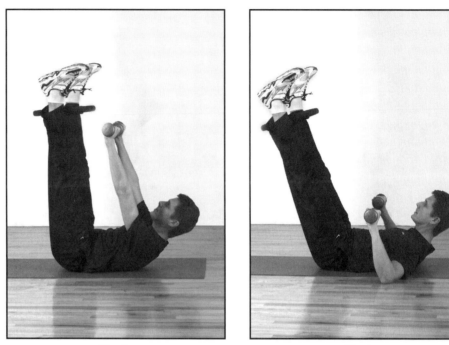

Step 2   Step 3

Step 1. Still lying on your back with the ring between your ankles and legs straight up in the air, take a weight in each hand. With your elbows out to the side and your forearms perpendicular to the floor, hold your weights up.

Step 2. As you exhale forcefully, squeeze the ring and curl up while pressing the weights up.

Step 3. As you inhale, bring your arms back to their starting position and lower your legs to an 80-degree angle but DO NOT LOWER FROM YOUR CURL.

Step 4. Repeat 8 times.

Exercise 8

EXTENDED LEG REVERSE CURL & PEC FLIES WITH RING AND HEAVY WEIGHTS

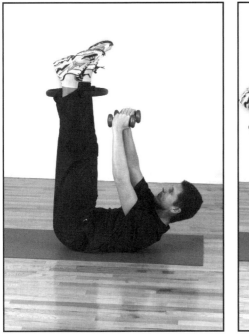

Step 2

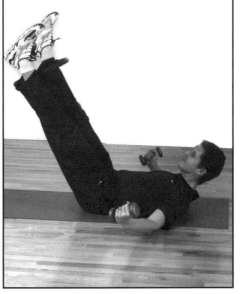

Step 3

This is the same exercise as #7 but with pectoral flies instead of a bench press.

Step 1. Still lying on your back, place the ring between your ankles and extend your legs straight up in the air at a 90-degree angle. Hold a weight in each hand, palms facing each other, with your arms out to the side and elbows slightly bent.

Step 2. Exhale, squeeze the ring, and curl up, arcing your arms up over your chest.

Step 3. Inhale, bring your arms back to their starting position, and lower your legs to an 80-degree angle but DO NOT LOWER FROM THE CURL.

Step 4. Repeat 8 times.

Strengthen the core muscles that are involved in trunk flexion. Intensify abdominal training by adding the ring and weights and involving more muscle groups in the same exercise.

TARGET MUSCLES:

Same as the previous exercise minus the *biceps* and *triceps* (arm) muscles.

TECHNIQUE TIPS:

Again, if you feel any discomfort in your lower back as you perform the exercise, stop and pull your knees into your chest.

Ab Series
Level 2

65

Back Series
Level 1

This sequence was designed to loosen up the spine as well as build shoulder muscle endurance. Use the forced exhalation breath to continually recruit the deepest abdominal layer (*transversus abdominis*) for support.

Exercise 1

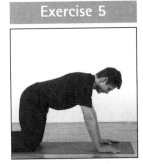

ARCH

Exercise 2

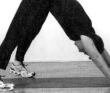

PUSH-UP HOLD

Exercise 3

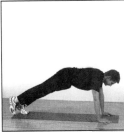

INVERTED V HOLD

Exercise 4

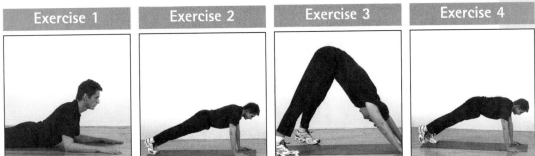

LEG LIFT IN A PUSH-UP HOLD

Exercise 5

CAT BACK STRETCH

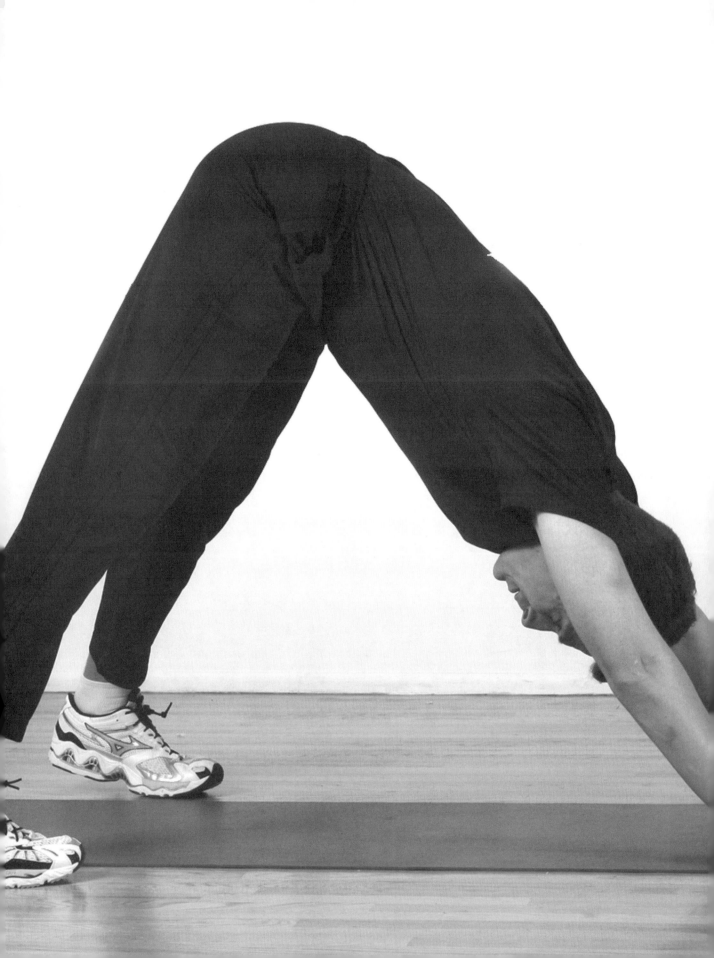

ARCH

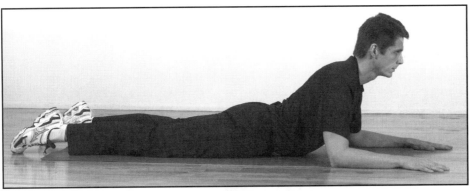

Step 1

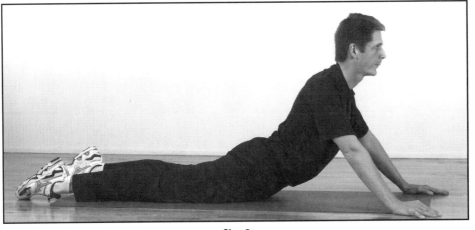

Step 2

Strengthen the abdominals and increase spine flexibility.

TARGET MUSCLES:

Internal and *external obliques* (intermediate abdominal layers), *iliopsoas* (hip flexor), *transversus abdominis* (deepest abdominal layer), *erector spinae* (spine), *multifidus* (back), and *quadratus lumborum* (lower back).

TECHNIQUE TIPS:

Don't compress your spine as you lift your chest up; instead, concentrate on keeping your ribcage stable, shoulders down, neck relaxed, and lower back long.

Step 1. Lie on your stomach with your forearms on the floor in front of you, palms down, and your legs straight on the floor, feet extended.

Step 2. As you exhale, press up with your arms, lengthen your waist, and lift your chest to come into a slight arch. Look straight ahead.

Step 3. Repeat 3 times, each time coming up a little higher.

Back Series
Level 1

GOAL:

Strengthen trunk and shoulder muscles.

TARGET MUSCLES:

Transversus abdominis (deepest abdominal layer), *diaphragm* (breathing muscle), adductor (inner thigh), *pelvic floor*, latisismuss dorsi (back muscle), *pectoralis* (chest), *deltoids* (shoulder), and *biceps* and *triceps* (arms).

TECHNIQUE TIPS:

Do not arch your back.

70

Exercise 2

PUSH-UP HOLD

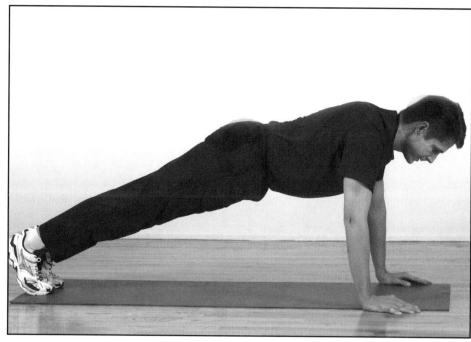

Step 2

Step 1. Still lying on your stomach with your legs straight, place your hands on the floor a little more than shoulder width apart.

Step 2. Press up onto the balls of the feet and lift your torso off the floor as if you are preparing to do a push-up.

Step 3. Exhale to contract your abdominals, lengthen the spine, and squeeze your butt and inner thigh muscles.

Step 4. Hold for 4 deep exhalations.

Exercise 3

INVERTED V HOLD

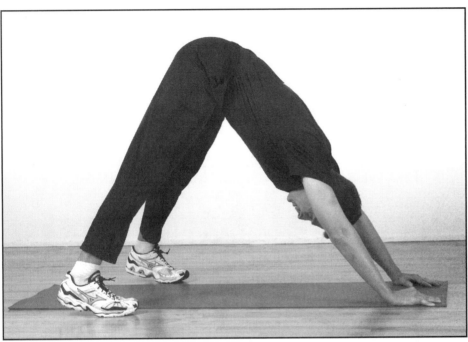

Step 3

Step 1. Come onto your hands and knees with your hands a little more than shoulder width apart and your knees about hip width apart. Your fingers should be turned toward each other.

Step 2. Inhale and tuck your toes under.

Step 3. As you exhale forcefully, tighten your abdominals, straighten your knees, and reach your hips and tailbone up to the ceiling. Keep the spine straight and long, and your shoulders down.

Step 4. Hold for 4 deep exhalations.

GOAL:
Strengthen the shoulders and arms while stabilizing the hips and spine.

TARGET MUSCLES:
Same as the previous exercise plus the *trapezius* (upper back), *biceps femoris* (hamstrings), *gastrocnemius* and *soleus* (calf) muscles.

TECHNIQUE TIPS:
Do not round or arch the back.

Back Series
Level 1

71

GOAL:

Strengthen the abdominals, shoulders, and hip extensors.

TARGET MUSCLES:

Same as exercise #2 plus the *quadratus lumborum* (lower back), *gluteus maximus* (butt), *medius*, and *minimus* (butt) muscles.

TECHNIQUE TIPS:

Be careful not to overextend your spine. Keep your neck relaxed and concentrate on keeping your shoulders and ribcage stabilized.

72

Exercise 4

LEG LIFT IN A PUSH-UP HOLD

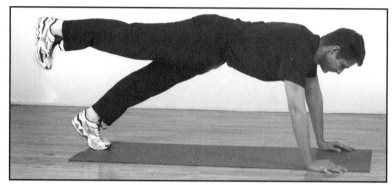

Step 3

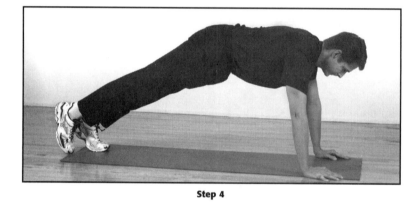

Step 4

Step 1. Lie on your stomach with your legs straight, place your hands on the floor a little wider than shoulder width apart.

Step 2. Press up onto the balls of the feet and lift your torso off the floor as if you are preparing to do a push-up.

Step 3. Pull your abdominals in toward your spine, lengthen the spine, and, as you exhale forcefully, lift your right leg up so that it makes a straight line with your back.

Step 4. Inhale as you lower your leg, touching the floor lightly.

Step 5. Repeat 4 times, then switch sides.

Exercise 5

CAT BACK STRETCH

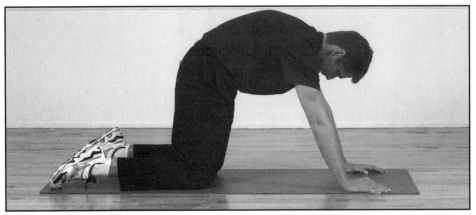

Step 2

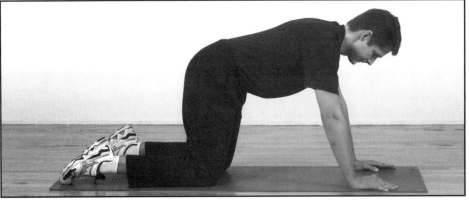

Step 3

GOAL:
Gain mobility in the spine and increase awareness of spinal movement.

TARGET MUSCLES:
Erector spinae (spine), *multifidus* (back), *quadratus lumborum* (lower back), *latissimus dorsi,* and lower *trapezius* (upper back).

TECHNIQUE TIPS:
Do not arch your back in Step 3.

Step 1. Come onto your hands and knees, with your knees directly under your hips. Keep your toes extended (that is, not curled under).

Step 2. Exhale forcefully and pull up through your *pelvic floor* and abdominals to round the spine.

Step 3. Inhale and straighten one vertebra at a time.

Step 4. Repeat 3 times. The last time, hold your back flat and tighten your abdominals.

Back Series
Level 1

Ab & Hip Series
Level 1

In this sequence, you add hip and shoulder exercises to the previous abdominal series.

Exercise 1	Exercise 2a	Exercise 2b	Exercise 3

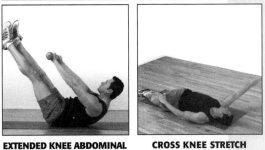

BENT KNEE ABDOMINAL CURL

BENT KNEE ABDOMINAL CURL & BENCH PRESS WITH HEAVY WEIGHTS OR ▸

EXTENDED KNEE ABDOMINAL CURL & BENCH PRESS WITH HEAVY WEIGHTS

CROSS KNEE STRETCH

Exercise 4	Exercise 5a	Exercise 5b	Exercise 6

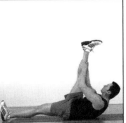
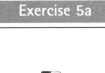
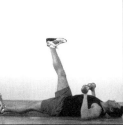
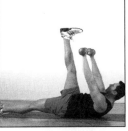
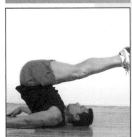

EXTENDED LEG ABDOMINAL CURL

EXTENDED LEG ABDOMINAL CURL & BENCH PRESS WITH HEAVY WEIGHTS OR ▸

LEG LIFT ABDOMINAL CURL & BENCH PRESS WITH HEAVY WEIGHT

OVERHEAD STRETCH

GOAL:

Stretch the spine and hips.

TARGET MUSCLES:

Transversus abdominis (deepest abdominal layer), *internal* and *external* obliques (intermediate abdominal layers), *rectus abdominis* (superficial abdominal layer),, *iliopsoas* (hip flexor), *biceps femoris* (hamstring), and *erector spinae* (spine) muscles.

TECHNIQUE TIPS:

Use a forced exhalation breath to initiate the stretch.

BENT KNEE ABDOMINAL CURL

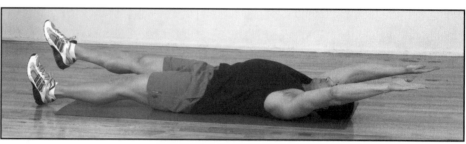

Step 1

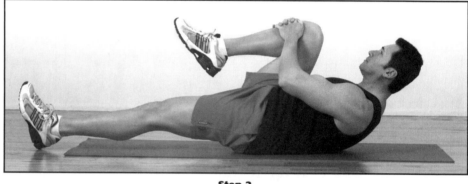

Step 2

Step 1. Lie on your back with your arms extended above your head and left leg straight on the floor. Your right leg should hover an inch or two above the floor. Lengthen through your spine by reaching your arms and legs away from each other.

Step 2. As you exhale forcefully, curl up just until your head and shoulders come off the floor, take hold of your right knee with your hands, pull it into your chest. Keep your left leg extended and pressed down for stability.

Step 3. As you inhale, lower into the starting position and reach your arms and legs away from each other.

Step 4. Repeat 4 times, then switch sides.

im
=X

BENT KNEE ABDOMINAL CURL & BENCH PRESS WITH HEAVY WEIGHTS

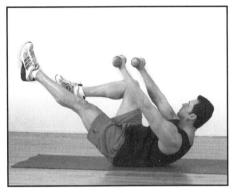

Step 2

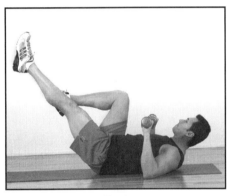

Step 3

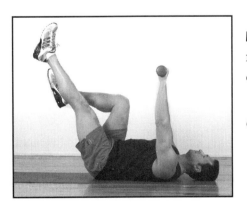

MODIFICATION

Step 1. Still lying on your back with your legs straight on the floor, take a weight in each hand. With your elbows out to the side and your forearms perpendicular to the floor, hold your weights up on either side of your chest, palms facing forward.

Step 2. As you exhale forcefully, bring your right knee into your chest, lift your left leg to a 45-degree angle, curl up, and press the weights up to the ceiling.

Step 3. As you inhale, lower your arms back to your starting position but do not lower from the curl. Keep the legs in position.

Step 4. Repeat 8 times, curling up a little higher each time, then switch sides.

MODIFICATION: If you are a beginner, try this exercise without the curl first.

OR

GOAL:
Strengthen the hip flexors, abdominal, and chest area while maintaining spinal alignment.

TARGET MUSCLES:
Transversus abdominis (deepest abdominal layer), *internal* and *external* obliques (intermediate abdominal layers), *rectus abdominis* (superficial abdominal layer), *pelvic floor*, *iliopsoas* (hip flexor), *quadriceps* (thigh), *latisimuss dorsi* (back muscle), *pectoralis* (chest), *deltoids* (shoulder), *biceps* and *triceps* (arms) muscles.

TECHNIQUE TIPS:
Use your exhale to tighten the lower abdominals to curl higher as you extend your arms.

Ab & Hip Series
Level 1

77

GOAL:

Strengthen the abdominal, hip, chest, and shoulder flexors.

TARGET MUSCLES:

Same as the previous exercise but with a focus on the *quadriceps* (thigh).

TECHNIQUE TIPS:

Before you add the bench press, practice pulling the knee in as you curl until it feels natural.

Exercise 2b

EXTENDED KNEE ABDOMINAL CURL & BENCH PRESS WITH HEAVY WEIGHTS

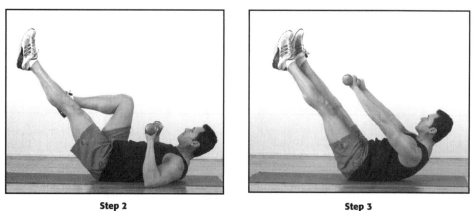

Step 2   Step 3

Step 1. Still lying on your back with your legs straight on the floor, take a weight in each hand. With your elbows out to the side and your forearms perpendicular to the floor, hold your weights up on either side of your chest, palms facing forward.

Step 2. As you exhale forcefully, bring your right knee into your chest, lift your left leg to a 45-degree angle, and curl up while you press the weights up to the ceiling.

Step 3. As you inhale, lower your upper body back to the starting position while you straighten your right leg to meet the left.

Step 4. Repeat 8 times, curling up a little higher each time, then switch sides.

im
=X

Exercise 3

CROSS KNEE STRETCH

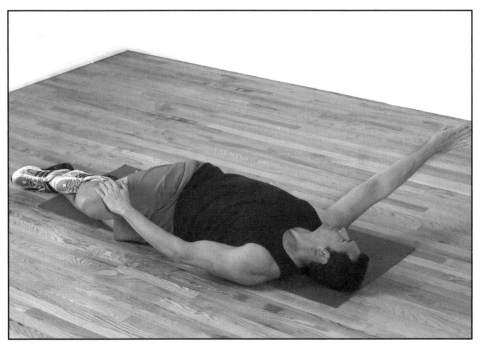

Step 3

Step 1. Lie on your back with your legs straight on the floor and your arms at your sides.

Step 2. Bring your right knee into your chest and pull it across your body to the left with your left hand.

Step 3. Place your right arm on a high diagonal, palm facing down as far as you can. Look toward your right hand.

Step 4. Exhale and stretch with both hands, then switch sides.

GOAL:
Stretch the lower spine and chest muscles.

TARGET MUSCLES:
Levatores, rotatores, erector spinae, quadratus lumborum, multifidus (back), and *internal* and *external obliques* (intermediate abdominal layers).

TECHNIQUE TIPS:
Reach through the fingertips of your upper hand to increase the flexibility at the shoulder.

Ab & Hip Series
Level 1

GOAL:

Strengthen the abdominal and hip flexors while increasing flexibility in the *biceps femoris* (hamstrings).

TARGET MUSCLES:

Transversus abdominis (deepest abdominal layer), *internal* and *external* obliques (intermediate abdominal layers), *rectus abdominis* (superficial abdominal layer),, *pelvic floor*, *iliopsoas* (hip flexor), *quadriceps* (thigh), and *biceps femoris* (hamstrings) muscles.

TECHNIQUE TIPS:

Do not compress your spine as you curl up.

80

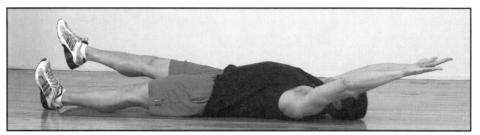

Exercise 4

EXTENDED LEG ABDOMINAL CURL

Step 1

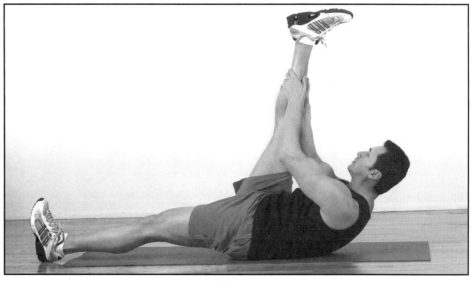

Step 2

Step 1. Lie on your back and reach your arms overhead and extend your right leg 3 to 5 inches off the floor.

Step 2. As you exhale, raise your right leg up to a perpendicular angle with the knee straight. Grab your right leg with your hands for a deeper stretch, if you prefer, and curl up until you feel your abdominals working.

Step 3. As you inhale, lower yourself slowly back to your starting position.

Step 4. Repeat 3 times, then switch sides.

Exercise 5a

EXTENDED LEG ABDOMINAL CURL & BENCH PRESS WITH HEAVY WEIGHTS

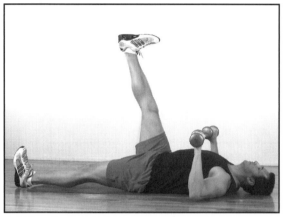

Step 1

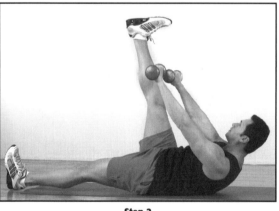

Step 2

Step 1. Lie on your back with your left leg on the floor and your right leg up in the air at a perpendicular angle. Flex both feet. Take a weight in each hand. With your elbows out to the side and your forearms perpendicular to the floor, hold your weights up on either side of your chest, palms facing forward.

Step 2. As you exhale forcefully, raise your right leg up to a perpendicular angle with the knee straight. Simultaneously, curl up until you feel your abdominals working and press the weights straight up to the ceiling.

Step 3. As you inhale, lower your torso slowly back to your starting position but hold your leg in position.

Step 4. Repeat 8 times, then switch sides.

OR

GOAL:
Stabilize the spine while increasing flexibility of the hamstrings.

TARGET MUSCLES:
Same as previous exercise plus *pectoralis* (chest), *deltoids* (shoulder), *biceps* and *triceps* (arms).

TECHNIQUE TIPS:
Keep the shoulders stabilized while you bench press.

Ab & Hip Series
Level 1

81

GOAL:

Improve range of motion at the hip while strengthening the flexors of the torso.

TARGET MUSCLES:

Same as the previous exercise.

TECHNIQUE TIPS:

Keep your leg straight and extended as you lift and lower it.

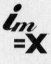

82

LEG LIFT ABDOMINAL CURL & BENCH PRESS WITH HEAVY WEIGHT

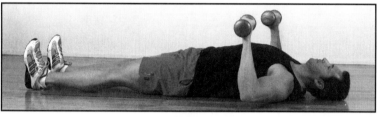

Step 1

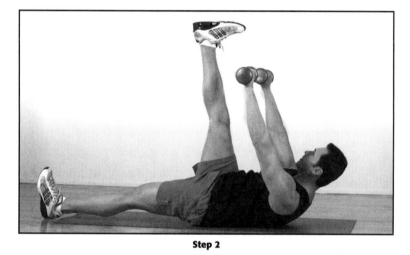

Step 2

Step 1. Lie on your back with your legs straight on the floor. Take a weight in each hand. With your elbows out to the side and your forearms perpendicular to the floor, hold your weights up on either side of your chest, palms facing forward.

Step 2. As you exhale forcefully, raise your right leg up to a perpendicular angle with the knee straight. Simultaneously, curl up until you feel your abdominals working and press the weights straight up to the ceiling.

Step 3. As you inhale, lower your torso slowly back to your starting position and lower your leg.

Step 4. Repeat 8 times, then switch sides.

OVERHEAD STRETCH

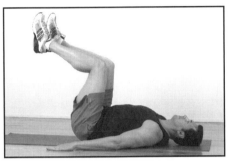

Step 1

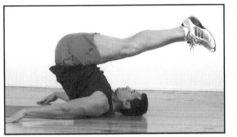

Step 2

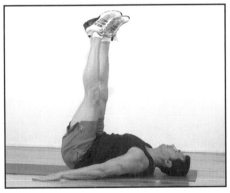

Step 3

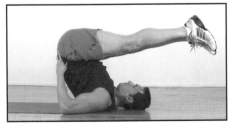

MODIFICATION

Step 1. Lie on your back with your arms on a low diagonal and bring your knees into your chest.

Step 2. As you exhale forcefully, straighten your legs and lift your buttocks to bring your legs over your head. Let your lower back stretch by allowing your legs to go as far as you feel comfortable. You may need to rock back and forth a few times to get your legs overhead.

Step 3. Inhale and roll down slowly, one vertebra at a time, until your back is on the ground and your legs are straight up in the air at a perpendicular angle.

Step 4. Repeat step 2 but this time stop when your legs are parallel to the floor.

Step 5. Repeat 5 times.

MODIFICATION: If it helps, you can use your hands to support your back in Step 2.

GOAL:

Strengthen the back, abdominal, and hip muscles. Increase spinal flexibility.

TARGET MUSCLES:

Transversus abdominis (deepest abdominal layer), *internal* and *external* obliques (intermediate abdominal layers), *rectus abdominis* (superficial abdominal layer),, *erector spinae* (spine), *multifidus* (back), *quadratus lumborum* (lower back), *latissimus dorsi*, lower *trapezius* (upper back), *pelvic floor*, *iliopsoas* (hip flexor), *quadriceps* (thigh), and *biceps femoris* (hamstrings) muscles.

TECHNIQUE TIPS:

Be sure to keep your neck relaxed and shoulders down. If you have

Ab & Hip Series Level 1

Back Series
Level 2

In Back Series Level 1, the exercises were performed in a static position. Here, we are adding movement for additional shoulder and upper back strength.

Exercise 1	Exercise 2	Exercise 3	Exercise 4

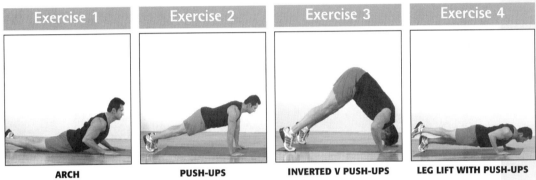

| ARCH | PUSH-UPS | INVERTED V PUSH-UPS | LEG LIFT WITH PUSH-UPS |

GOAL:

Increase flexibility in the back.

TARGET MUSCLES:

Transversus abdominis (deepest abdominal layer), *internal* and *external obliques* (intermediate abdominal layers), *iliopsoas* (hip flexor), *erector spinae* (spine), *levatores, rotatores, multifidus* (back), and *quadratus lumborum* (lower back) muscles.

TECHNIQUE TIPS:

Don't compress your spine as you lift your chest up; instead, concentrate on keeping your ribcage stable, shoulders down, and neck relaxed.

ARCH

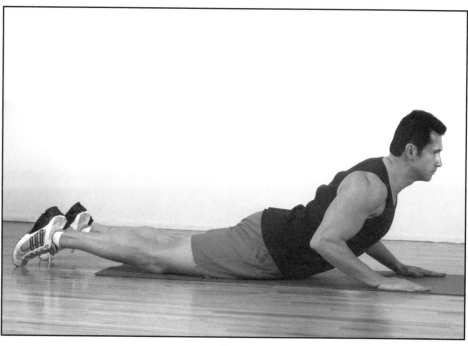

Step 2

Step 1. Lie on your stomach with your arms stretched out in front of you, palms down, and your legs straight on the floor.

Step 2. As you exhale, press up, lengthening your waist, as you come into a slight arch.

Step 3. Repeat 3 times, each time coming up a little higher.

PUSH-UPS

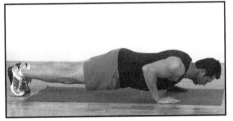

Step 2

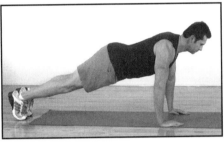

Step 3

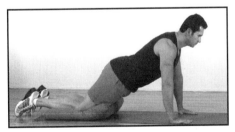

MODIFICATION #1

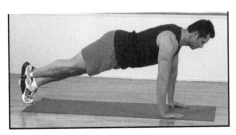

MODIFICATION #2

Step 1. Still lying on your stomach with your legs straight, place your hands on the floor a little wider than shoulder width apart. Your fingers should face in toward each other.

Step 2. Press up onto the balls of the feet and lift your torso off the floor to get into a push-up position.

Step 3. Inhale, pull your abdominals in toward your spine, and lower yourself toward the floor.

Step 4. As you exhale, contract your abdominals and squeeze your legs tight as you press up.

Step 5. Repeat 10 to 20 times.

MODIFICATION #1: If you are a beginner, in step 2, press up onto the knees instead of the balls of your feet. Place a pillow under your knees to protect them, and keep your lower leg on the floor.

MODIFICATION #2: If you would like to make the exercise a little tougher, in step 2, cross your left foot over your right ankle and shift your weight to the right foot. Push up 5 to 10 times on the right, then switch sides.

GOAL:
Strengthen the trunk and shoulders.

TARGET MUSCLES:
Transversus abdominis (deepest abdominal layer), *diaphragm* (breathing muscle), *adductors* (inner thigh), *pelvic floor*, *latisimuss dorsi*(upper back), *pectoralis* (chest), *rhomboids*, serratus anterior, *deltoids* (shoulder), and *biceps* and *triceps* (arms).

TECHNIQUE TIPS:
Do not arch your back.

Back Series
Level 2

GOAL:

Strengthen the shoulders and arms while stabilizing the hips and spine.

TARGET MUSCLES:

Same as the previous exercise plus the *trapezius* (upper back), *biceps femoris* (hamstrings), *gastrocnemius* and *soleus* (calf) muscles and focusing on the *latissimus dorsi* (upper back).

TECHNIQUE TIPS:

Do not round or arch the back.

im =X

88

INVERTED V PUSH-UPS

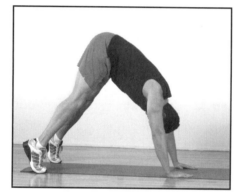

Step 1

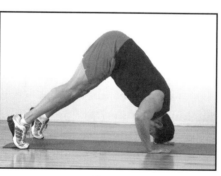

Step 2

Step 3

Step 1. Come onto your hands and knees with your hands a little more than shoulder width apart and your knees about hip width apart. Your fingers should face in toward each other.

Step 2. As you exhale forcefully, tighten your abs, straighten your knees, and reach your hips and tailbone up to the ceiling. Keep the spine straight and long, and your shoulders down.

Step 3. Inhale, bend your arms, and lower the top of your head towards the floor.

Step 4. Exhale, contract your abdominals, straighten your arms, and press back to the V hold.

Step 5. Repeat 10 times.

Exercise 4

LEG LIFT WITH PUSH-UPS

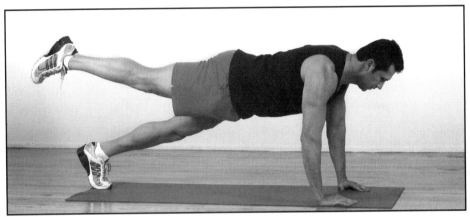

Step 2

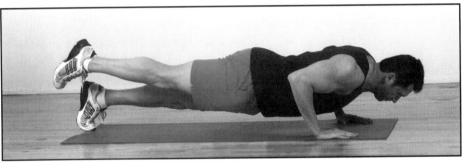

Step 3

TARGET MUSCLES:
Same as exercise #2 but adding the *quadratus lumborum* (lower back), and *gluteal* (butt) muscles.

TECHNIQUE TIPS:
Use your abdominals to initiate the movement, but you should also feel your *latissimus dorsi* (upper back) working as you press up.

Step 1. Lie on your stomach with your legs straight, place your hands on the floor a little wider than shoulder width apart and tuck your toes under.

Step 2. As you exhale, push up and lift your right leg to approximately a 45-degree angle.

Step 3. Keep your abdominals tight and spine long as you inhale and lower yourself toward the floor, lowering your leg to the floor as well.

Step 4. Exhale as you straighten your arms to push back up and lift your leg back up.

Step 5. Repeat 8 times, then switch sides.

Back Series
Level 2

89

Ab & Hip Series
Level 2

This sequence consists of more challenging movements because you are now moving your arms and legs simultaneously. You should focus on stabilizing your hips and shoulders so that you are working with control, rather than momentum. This will also increase your muscle endurance.

Exercise 1a	Exercise 1b	Exercise 2a	Exercise 2b

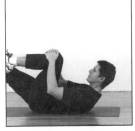

ABDOMINAL CURL KNEE CHANGES OR ▸

ABDOMINAL CURL LEG CHANGES

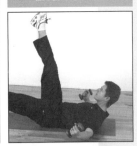

ABDOMINAL CURL KNEE CHANGES & PEC FLIES WITH LIGHT WEIGHTS OR ▸

ABDOMINAL CURL LEG CHANGES & PEC FLIES WITH LIGHT WEIGHTS

Exercise 3a	Exercise 3b	Exercise 4a	Exercise 4b

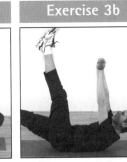

ABDOMINAL CURL KNEE CHANGES & BENCH PRESS WITH HEAVY WEIGHTS OR ▸

ABDOMINAL CURL LEG CHANGES & BENCH PRESS WITH HEAVY WEIGHTS

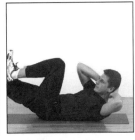

OBLIQUE CURL KNEE CHANGES OR ▸

OBLIQUE CURL LEG CHANGES

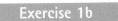

91

GOAL:

Strengthen the abdominals and increase flexibility in the legs and hips.

TARGET MUSCLES:

Transversus abdominis (deepest abdominal layer), *internal* and *external obliques* (intermediate abdominal layers), *pelvic floor, iliopsoas* (hip flexor), *biceps femoris* (hamstrings), and *quadriceps* (thigh) muscles.

TECHNIQUE TIPS:

Be sure not to jut your head forward as you curl up. Instead, keep your neck relaxed and your shoulders still.

92

ABDOMINAL CURL KNEE CHANGES

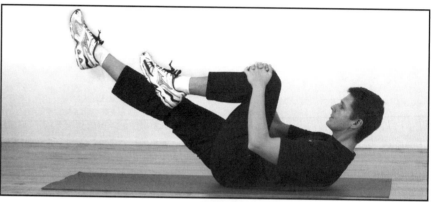

Step 2

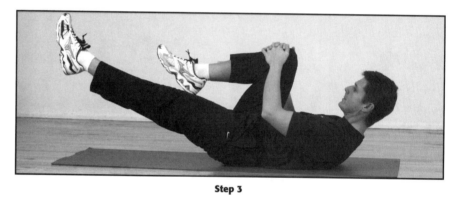

Step 3

Step 1. Lie on your back with your legs straight on the floor and arms by your sides. Keep your toes extended.

Step 2. Pull your left knee into your chest and lift your left leg off the floor. At the same time, exhale forcefully and curl up. Your left foot should line up with your right knee.

Step 3. Exhale and stretch the right knee into your chest while straightening your right leg several inches off the floor. DO NOT LOWER FROM THE CURL.

Step 4. Repeat 8 times, making sure to exhale each time you change knees.

OR

ABDOMINAL CURL LEG CHANGES

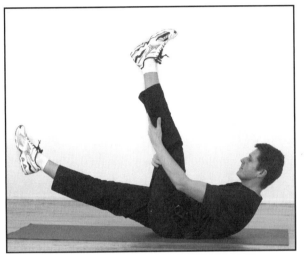

Step 2

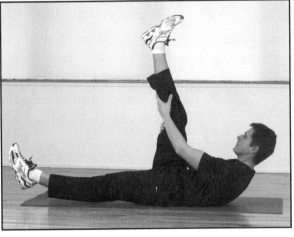

Step 3

This is the same as exercise #1a but with your legs straight.

Step 1. Lie on your back with your legs straight on the floor and arms by your sides.

Step 2. Raise your left leg straight up in the air until it is perpendicular to the floor, grabbing it with your hands for a stretch, and lift your right leg several inches off the floor. At the same time, exhale forcefully and curl up until you feel your abdominals working.

Step 3. Inhale, then exhale forcefully and change legs, raising the right leg to a perpendicular angle and lowering your left leg until it is an inch or two off the floor. DO NOT LOWER FROM THE CURL.

Step 4. Repeat 8 times, making sure to exhale each time you change legs.

GOAL:
Strengthen the abdominal wall and hip flexors while increasing hamstring flexibility.

TARGET MUSCLES:
Same as the previous exercise.

TECHNIQUE TIPS:
Again, make sure you are working from your arms and abdominals as you stretch your legs instead of pulling from your neck and shoulders.

Ab & Hip Series
Level 2

GOAL:

Build endurance in the upper abdominal and chest muscles.

TARGET MUSCLES:

Same as previous exercise plus *pectoralis* (chest), *deltoids* (shoulder), *biceps* and *triceps* (arms).

TECHNIQUE TIPS:

You are basically holding an abdominal curl and then increasing the curl by 3 inches as the arms come together.

94

ABDOMINAL CURL KNEE CHANGES & PEC FLIES WITH LIGHT WEIGHTS

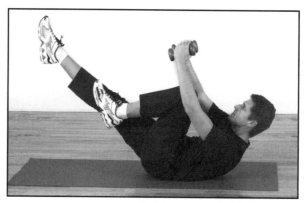

Step 2

Step 1. Still lying on your back with your legs straight on the floor, take a weight in each hand, palms facing each other, with your arms out to the side and elbows slightly bent.

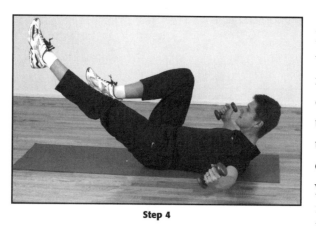

Step 4

Step 2. As you exhale forcefully, bring your left knee into your chest, lift your right leg several inches off the floor, and curl up. At the same time, arc your arms up until they are directly over your chest, keeping your elbows rounded, as if you were hugging a big tree.

Step 3. As you inhale, lower your arms back to your starting position but stay curled up.

Step 4. As you exhale, switch knees, curl up 3 inches higher, arc your arms in again, then lower.

Step 5. Repeat 8 times on each side.

OR

ABDOMINAL CURL LEG CHANGES & PEC FLIES WITH LIGHT WEIGHTS

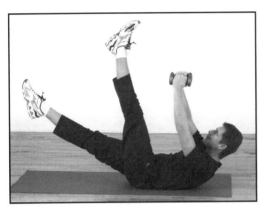

Step 2

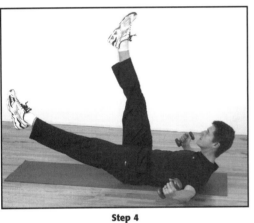

Step 4

Step 1. Still lying on your back with your legs straight on the floor, take a weight in each hand, palms facing each other, with your arms out to the side and elbows slightly bent.

Step 2. As you exhale, raise your left leg straight up until it is perpendicular to the floor with your right leg several inches off the floor. At the same time, curl up and arc your arms up over your chest, keeping your elbows rounded, as if you were hugging a big tree.

Step 3. As you inhale, lower your arms but stay curled up and keep your legs in place.

Step 4. As you exhale, switch legs, curl up an additional 3 inches, arc your arms up, then lower.

Step 5. Repeat 8 times on each side.

GOAL:
Strengthen the abdominal and chest muscles while stretching the *biceps femoris* (hamstrings).

TARGET MUSCLES:
Same as the previous exercise but with more emphasis on the chest muscles.

Ab & Hip Series
Level 2

95

Exercise 3a

ABDOMINAL CURL KNEE CHANGES & BENCH PRESS WITH HEAVY WEIGHTS

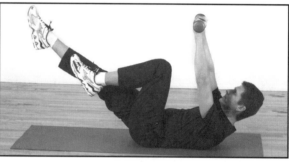

Step 2

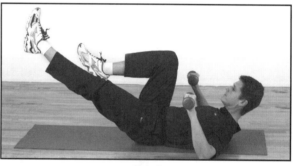

Step 4

Step 1. Still lying on your back with your legs straight on the floor, take a weight in each hand. With your elbows out to the side and your forearms perpendicular to the floor, hold your weights up on either side of your chest, palms facing forward.

Step 2. As you exhale forcefully, bring your left knee into your chest, lift your right leg several inches off the floor, and curl up until you feel your abdominals working. At the same time, press your arms straight up to the ceiling.

Step 3. As you inhale, lower your arms but stay curled up.

Step 4. As you exhale, switch knees, curl up 3 additional inches as you extend your arms, then lower.

Step 5. Repeat 8 times on each side.

OR

ABDOMINAL CURL LEG CHANGES & BENCH PRESS WITH HEAVY WEIGHTS

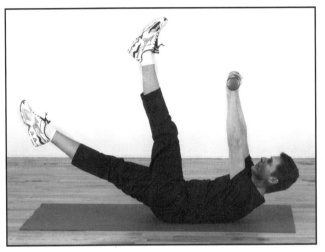

Step 2

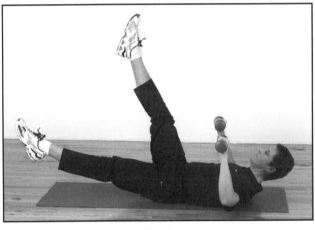

Step 4

Step 1. Still lying on your back with your legs straight on the floor, take a weight in each hand. With your elbows out to the side and your forearms perpendicular to the floor, hold your weights up on either side of your chest, palms facing forward.

Step 2. As you exhale, raise your left leg straight up in the air until it is perpendicular to the floor, lift your right leg several inches off the floor, and curl up until you feel your abdominals working. At the same time, press your arms straight up to the ceiling.

Step 3. As you inhale, lower your arms but stay curled up.

Step 4. As you exhale, switch legs, curl up 3 additional inches as you extend your arms, then lower.

Step 5. Repeat 8 times on each side.

GOAL:
Strengthen the abdominal and hip muscles while increasing flexibility in the *biceps femoris* (hamstrings).

TARGET MUSCLES:
Transversus abdominis (deepest abdominal layer), *internal* and *external obliques* (intermediate abdominal layers), *rectus abdominis* (superficial abdominal layer), *pelvic floor, iliopsoas* (hip flexor), *biceps femoris* (hamstrings), *latissimus dorsi* (upper back), *pectoralis* (chest), and *deltoids* (shoulder) muscles.

Ab & Hip Series
Level 2

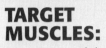

Strengthen the *internal* and *external obliques* (intermediate abdominal layers).

TARGET MUSCLES:

Same as exercise #1a but with a stronger emphasis on strengthening the *oblique* abdominals.

TECHNIQUE TIPS:

Bring your elbow towards the opposite knee by rotating your torso rather than just moving the arm; this will strengthen your *oblique* abdominals.

98

Exercise 4a

OBLIQUE CURL KNEE CHANGES

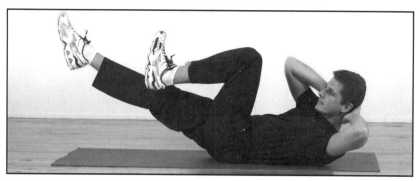

Step 2

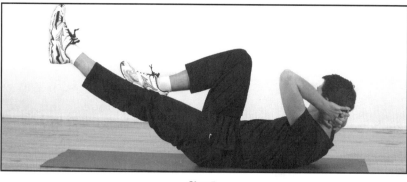

Step 3

Step 1. Still lying on your back with your legs straight on the floor, place your hands behind your head to support your neck.

Step 2. As you exhale forcefully, bring your left knee into your chest, lift your left leg 3 to 5 inches off the floor, and curl up with your right elbow toward your left knee.

Step 3. As you exhale again, switch knees, rotating your torso to reach your left elbow toward the right knee. Stay curled up as you alternate sides.

Step 4. Repeat 8 times.

OR

OBLIQUE CURL LEG CHANGES

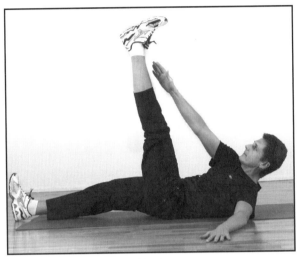

Step 2

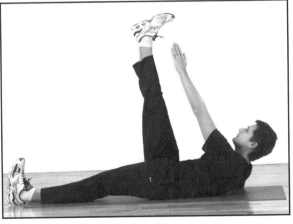

Step 3

Step 1. Still lying on your back with your legs straight on the floor, place your right hand, palm up, on a high diagonal and your left hand, palm down, on a low diagonal.

Step 2. As you exhale forcefully, raise your left leg straight up in the air until it is perpendicular to the floor, and curl up. At the same time, reach your right arm across your body toward your left knee.

Step 3. As you exhale again, switch legs, and reach your left arm across towards your right leg. Stay curled up as you alternate sides.

Step 4. Repeat 8 times on each side.

GOAL:
Strengthen the *oblique* abdominals and stretch the shoulder joint and hamstrings.

TARGET MUSCLES:
Same as exercise #1b but with a stronger emphasis on strengthening the *oblique* abdominals.

Ab & Hip Series
Level 2

Lateral Moves

This strengthens the muscles that produce lateral motion in the hips and spine while developing flexibility in the lumbar spine and legs. This helps you lunge for the ball when you're playing tennis, racquetball, or other sports.

NOTE: You will want to do this entire sequence on one side, and then switch to the other side.

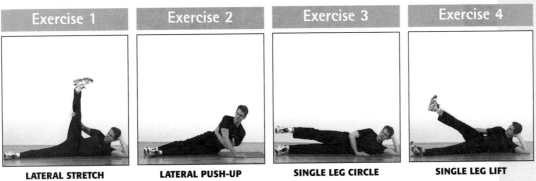

Exercise 1	Exercise 2	Exercise 3	Exercise 4
LATERAL STRETCH	LATERAL PUSH-UP	SINGLE LEG CIRCLE	SINGLE LEG LIFT

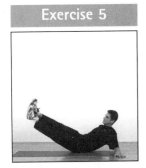

Exercise 5

DOUBLE LEG LIFT

Increase flexibility in the hip and legs.

TECHNIQUE TIPS:

Do not move your spine or hips during this stretch.

LATERAL STRETCH

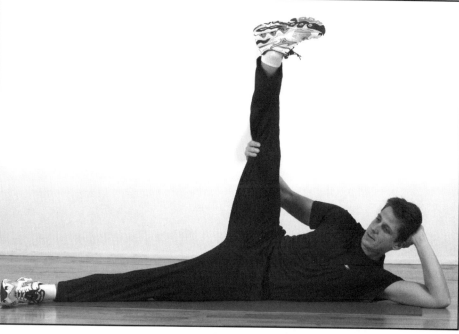

Step 3

Step 1. Lie on your left side with your legs straight but angled in front of your body. Place your left hand at your head, your left hand on the floor in front of your ribcage.

Step 2. Turn your right leg so that your knee is pointed up. Then, exhale and lift your right leg as high as you can without moving your hip. Be sure to keep the leg straight.

Step 3. Take hold of your leg with your right hand, tighten your abdominal and pelvic muscles, and pull your leg further toward yourself for a stretch. Hold for 10 seconds, then lower.

Exercise 2

LATERAL PUSH-UP

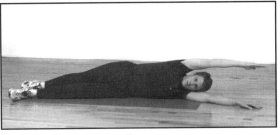

Step 1

Step 1. Lying on your left side, scissor your legs on the floor so that the top leg is behind and bottom leg is front.

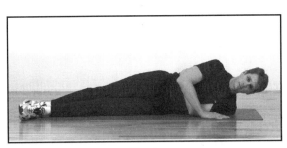

Step 2

Step 2. Then place your right hand down in front of your ribcage and your left hand at your ribcage. Exhale and straighten your right arm to push your torso up.

Step 3. As you inhale, bend your right arm to lower yourself slowly down.

Step 4. Repeat 10 times.

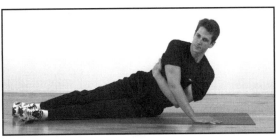

Step 3

GOAL:

Strengthen the oblique abdominals, hip extensors, hip flexors, *biceps* and *triceps* (arm), and chest muscles.

TARGET MUSCLES:

Transversus abdominis (deepest abdominal layer), *diaphragm* (breathing muscle), *internal* and *external obliques* (intermediate abdominal layers), *pelvic floor*, *iliopsoas* (hip flexor), *quadratus lumborum* (lower back), *biceps* and *triceps* (arm), and *pectoralis* (chest) muscles.

TECHNIQUE TIPS:

If you find it easier, you can keep your legs stacked one on top of the other with your feet together.

Lateral Moves

103

GOAL:

Strengthen and increase range of motion in the hips.

TARGET MUSCLES:

Transversus abdominis (deepest abdominal layer), *diaphragm* (breathing muscle), *pelvic floor*, *iliopsoas* (hip flexor), *quadratus lumborum* (lower back), *biceps femoris* (hamstrings), *quadriceps* (thigh), and *gluteal* (butt) muscles.

TECHNIQUE TIPS:

Anchor your hips and spine as you increase the size of the circle.

Exercise 3

SINGLE LEG CIRCLE

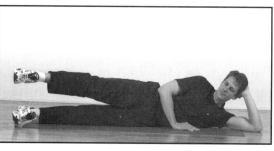

Step 1

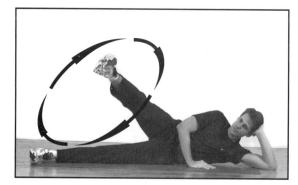

Step 2

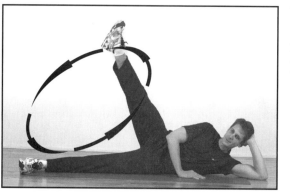

Step 3

Step 1. Still lying on your left side with your legs straight, your left hand supporting your head, and your right hand on the floor by your ribcage, exhale and make a circle with your right leg without moving your hips and lower back.

Step 2. Make the circles larger with each exhale to challenge your range of motion.

Step 3. Repeat 10 times and then reverse directions. Again, progress from small to larger circles. Be sure not to move your hips and lower back.

SINGLE LEG LIFT

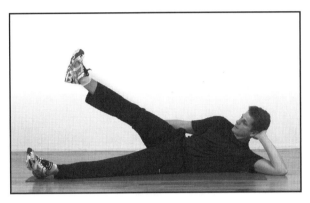

Step 2

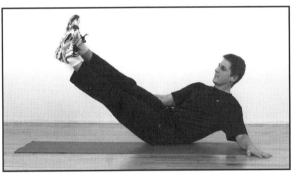

Step 3

Step 1. Still lying on your left side with your legs straight, put your left hand on the ground and come up on to your forearm. With your right hand on your hip, roll back slightly onto your left buttock.

Step 2. Tighten the abdominals and lift your top leg up to about a 45-degree angle.

Step 3. Exhale forcefully, lift your bottom leg up to the top leg, and squeeze your inner thighs together.

Step 4. Lower your bottom leg down as you inhale.

Step 5. Repeat 10 times.

GOAL:

Strengthen the abdominal, hip flexor, and thigh muscles.

TARGET MUSCLES:

Transversus abdominis (deepest abdominal layer), *internal* and *external* obliques (intermediate abdominal layers), *rectus abdominis* (superficial abdominal layer), *pelvic floor, iliopsoas* (hip flexor), *quadratus lumborum* (lower back), *biceps femoris* (hamstrings), *quadriceps* (thigh), and *gluteal* (butt) muscles.

TECHNIQUE TIPS:

Try not to move your head forward as you lift your leg. If you find it easier, you can hold your top leg with your left hand.

Lateral Moves

GOAL:

Strengthen the abdominals and hip flexors.

TARGET MUSCLES:

Same as the previous exercise with added intensity for the *oblique* abdominals and hip flexors.

TECHNIQUE TIPS:

If you feel any pain in your back, make sure you are using your forced exhalation breath to initiate the movement. If you still feel pain, STOP and skip this exercise.

106

DOUBLE LEG LIFT

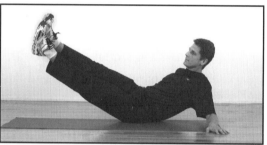

Step 2

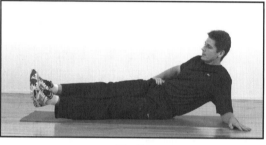

Step 3

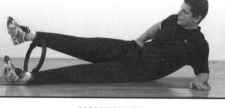

MODIFICATION

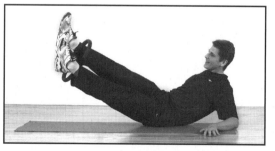

MODIFICATION

This is the same exercise as #4 but both legs are moving.

Step 1. Still lying on your left side with your legs straight, put your left hand on the ground and come up on to your forearm. With your right hand on your hip, roll back slightly onto your left buttock.

Step 2. Exhale, tighten your abdominals, squeeze your inner thighs, and lift both legs up to about a 45-degree angle.

Step 3. Lower both legs down briefly, before lifting them again.

Step 4. Repeat 10 times.

MODIFICATION: For increased difficulty, squeeze the ring between your ankles as you lift the legs up and down.

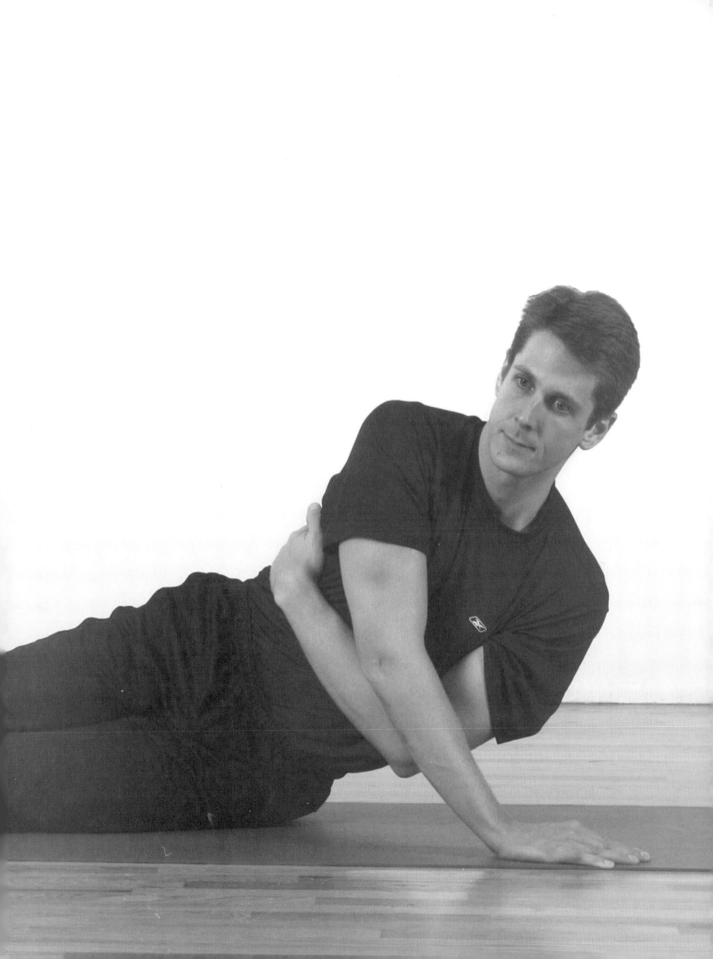

Spine Stabilizer Series

The following exercises challenge not only core strength but also spine mobility. In this first exercise, you will be required to apply all of the IM=X fundamentals: elongation, forced exhalation, and stabilization.

Exercise 1

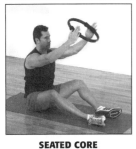

SEATED CORE
RECRUITMENT WITH RING

Exercise 2

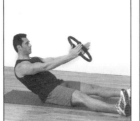

SPINE CURL WITH RING

Exercise 3

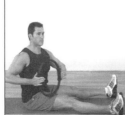

SPINE ROTATION WITH RING

Exercise 4

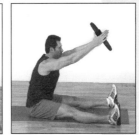

SPINE REACH WITH RING

Exercise 5

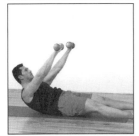

SPINE CURL & BENCH
PRESS WITH HEAVY
WEIGHTS

GOAL:

Improve skeletal alignment and create isometric strength in all of your torso muscles.

TARGET MUSCLES:

Transversus abdominis (deepest abdominal layer), *internal* and *external obliques* (deeper abdominal layers), *diaphragm* (breathing muscle), *pelvic floor*, *iliopsoas* (hip flexor), *erector spinae* (spine), *multifidus* (back), *quadratus lumborum* (lower back), *latissimus dorsi*, lower *trapezius* (upper back), *deltoids* (shoulder), and *pectoralis* (chest) muscles.

TECHNIQUE TIPS:

Do not lift your shoulders; instead, use your *latissimus dorsi* (upper back) to lift upward.

SEATED CORE RECRUITMENT WITH RING

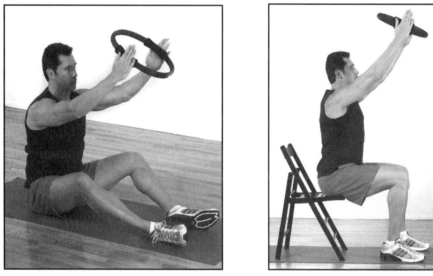

Step 2   MODIFICATION

Step 1. Sit on the floor with your legs in a diamond shape or shoulder width apart, and hold the ring in front of you with both hands.

Step 2. Reach your arms up and forward and lengthen your spine.

Step 3. Exhale, tighten your *pelvic floor*, abdominal and upper back muscles as you press lightly against the ring.

Step 4. Repeat 4 times, concentrating on elongating the back and deepening the muscle core effort each time.

MODIFICATION: You can also sit on the edge of a chair for this exercise.

SPINE CURL WITH RING

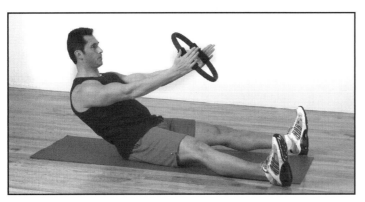

Step 1

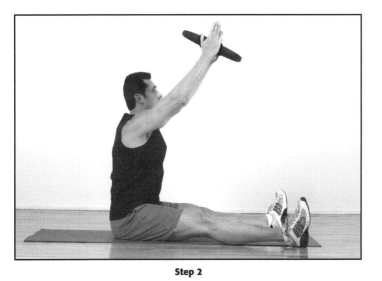

Step 2

GOAL:
Improve mobility in the lower back.

TARGET MUSCLES:
Same as the previous exercise.

TECHNIQUE TIPS:
Keep your shoulders down and neck relaxed. Use the ring to engage your upper back and chest muscles rather than your *biceps* and neck.

Step 1. Still sitting on the floor with your legs in a diamond or shoulder width apart, exhale forcefully, tighten your core muscles as instructed in the previous exercise, roll back halfway down slowly, and round your back, pressing lightly against the ring.

Step 2. Inhale, roll back up to your starting position, lengthen the spine, and reach up. Keep the shoulders down and waist long.

Step 3. Repeat 8 times.

Spine Stabilizer Series

GOAL:

Increase rotational flexibility in the spine.

TARGET MUSCLES:

Same as the previous exercise but with a focus on strengthening the muscles that rotate the spine—*transversus abdominis* (deepest abdominal layer), *internal* and *external obliques* (intermediate abdominal layers), *multifidus* and *rotatores* (back) muscles.

TECHNIQUE TIPS:

Use your oblique abdominals and *latissimus dorsi* (upper back) to initiate the movement. Keep your neck relaxed and shoulders down as you lengthen your spine and pelvis.

Exercise 3

SPINE ROTATION WITH RING

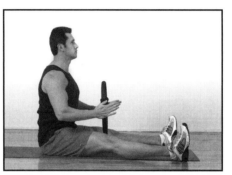

Step 1

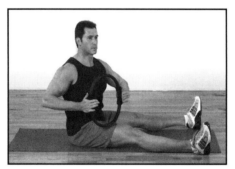

Step 2

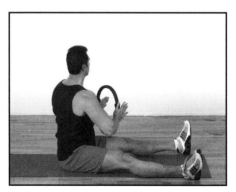

Step 4

Step 1. Still sitting, lengthen your spine, and place the ring in front of your chest.

Step 2. Exhale and press lightly against the ring to rotate your torso to the right.

Step 3. Inhale, and lengthen the spine.

Step 4. Exhale forcefully, and rotate to the left.

Step 5. Repeat 4 times in each direction.

im =X

Exercise 4

SPINE REACH WITH RING

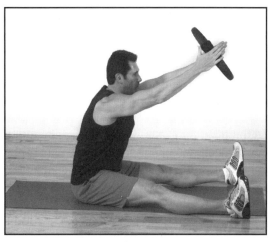

Step 2

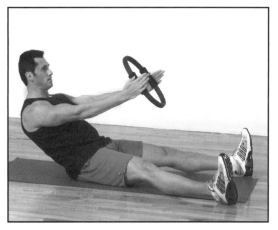

Step 3

Step 1. Sitting slightly forward on the pelvis with your legs stretched out in front of you, reach your ring overhead.

Step 2. Exhale forcefully, tighten your abdominals, and hinge forward slightly at the hips as you press lightly against the ring. Reach forward with your spine and ring.

Step 3. Roll as far down as you can and then return slowly to the seated position.

Step 4. Repeat 4 times slowly.

GOAL:
Increase flexibility in the spine, hips, and hamstrings.

TARGET MUSCLES:
Same as exercise #2.

TECHNIQUE TIPS:
Try not to tuck the hips under as you reach forward but rather lengthen your lower back and hinge forward at the hips.

Spine Stabilizer Series

GOAL:

Strengthen the abdominal, back, and shoulder muscles.

TARGET MUSCLES:

Same as exercise #3 but with a focus on the *deltoids* (shoulder), upper *trapezius* (upper back), and *erector spinae* (spine) muscles.

TECHNIQUE TIPS:

Be sure to keep your legs straight.

Exercise 5

SPINE CURL & BENCH PRESS WITH HEAVY WEIGHTS

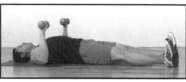

Step 1

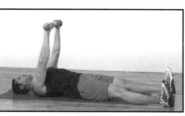

Step 2

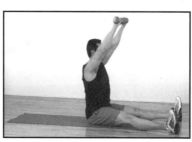

Step 3

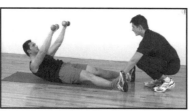

MODIFICATION #1

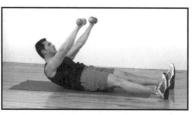

MODIFICATION #2

Step 1. Lie on your back with your legs straight on the floor, feet flexed. Take a weight in each hand. With your elbows out to the side and your forearms perpendicular to the floor, hold your weights up on either side of your chest, palms facing forward.

Step 2. Exhale forcefully, tighten your abdominals, and press the weights straight up to the ceiling, then lower. Repeat 5 times.

Step 3. On the final repetition, roll all the way up to a sitting position while pressing the weights straight up in the air.

Step 4. Lengthen the spine by reaching your arms up as far as you can before rolling down slowly.

Step 5. Repeat for 5 sets.

MODIFICATION #1: You may need to hook your legs on something, or have a partner hold them down, when you roll up. Be sure to keep your legs straight.

MODIFICATION #2: If you are a beginner, simply curl up as far as you can and hold, instead of rolling all the way to a sitting position.

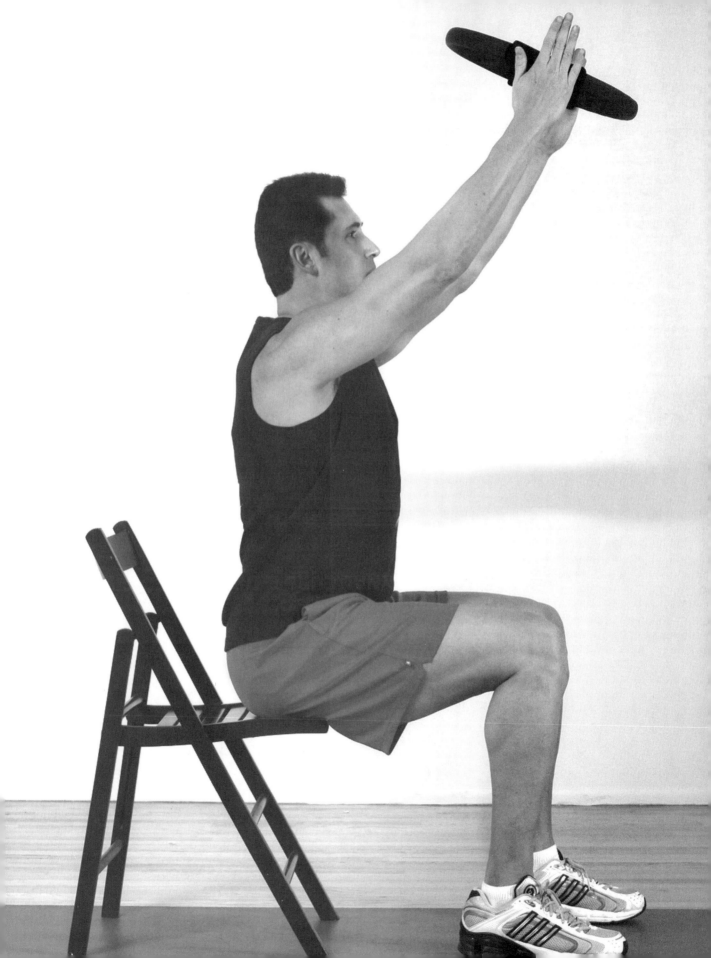

Chapter 13

Stretch Series
Level 2

Use this series to increase flexibility in your hip and leg muscles. Continue to focus on spine stabilization as you increase the range of the stretch.

Exercise 1	Exercise 2	Exercise 3	Exercise 4

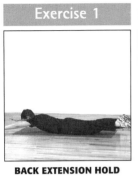

BACK EXTENSION HOLD

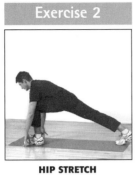

HIP STRETCH

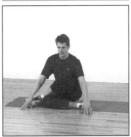

GLUTEAL STRETCH

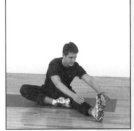

HAMSTRING STRETCH

Exercise 5

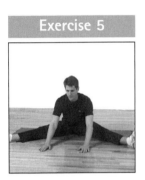

ADDUCTOR STRETCH

GOAL:

Develop endurance in the extensor muscles of the back and hips.

TARGET MUSCLES:

Transversus abdominis (deepest abdominal layer), *erector spinae* (spine), *levatores, rotatores, multifidus* (back), and *quadratus lumborum* (lower back) muscles.

TECHNIQUE TIPS:

Your abdominals and back muscles should be working together with the forced exhalation breath to hold the position.

im=X

Exercise 1

BACK EXTENSION HOLD

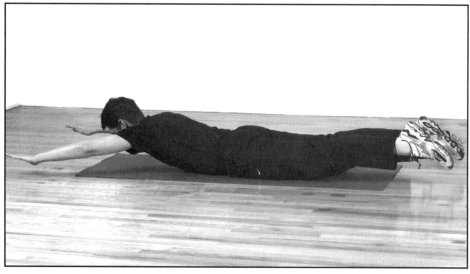

Step 2

Step 1. Lie on your stomach with your arms straight on the floor above your head and your legs straight.

Step 2. Exhale forcefully, tighten your abdominals, and raise your arms and legs off the mat a couple of inches.

Step 3. Hold for 4 deep exhalations.

Note: Do exercises #2 through #5 on one side, then repeat them all on the other side.

Exercise 2

HIP STRETCH

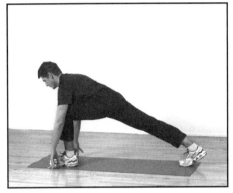

Step 1

Step 1. From your lying position, press your upper body up with hands on the floor and bring your left foot in front of you until your left knee makes a 90-degree angle with your right leg extended behind you.

Step 2. Exhale forcefully, lengthen your spine, and stretch.

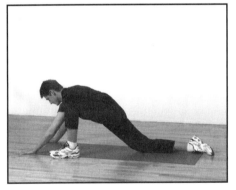

Step 3

Step 3. Rotate your front leg so that your knee faces out (externally rotate your left leg), and lower your back knee to the floor.

Step 4. Hold for 4 deep exhalations.

GOAL:

To stretch the hip flexors.

TARGET MUSCLES:

Iliopsoas (hip flexor), *biceps femoris* (hamstrings), and other muscles of your hips and legs.

TECHNIQUE TIPS:

Make sure your left knee is at a right angle directly over your toes for proper alignment.

Stretch Series
Level 2

GOAL:

To stretch the *gluteal* (butt) muscles.

TARGET MUSCLES:

Gluteus maximus (butt), *medius* (butt), *minimus* (butt), *quadratus lumborum* (lower back) and other muscles of the legs and hips while contracting the *pelvic floor*.

TECHNIQUE TIPS:

Lengthen your spine and tighten your abdominals as you reach forward.

GLUTEAL STRETCH

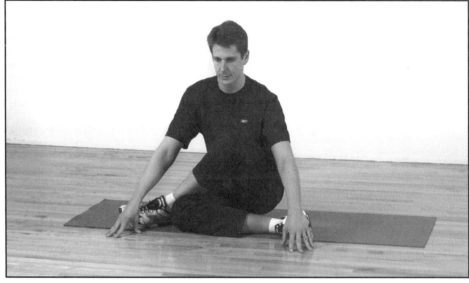

Step 2

Step 1. From the lunge position you were using for your hip stretch, fold your back leg underneath you and sit back.

Step 2. Reach your arms forward as far as you can to stretch in your *gluteal* muscles. Keep your back straight.

Step 3. Hold for 4 deep exhalations, reaching further each time.

im
=X

Exercise 4

HAMSTRING STRETCH

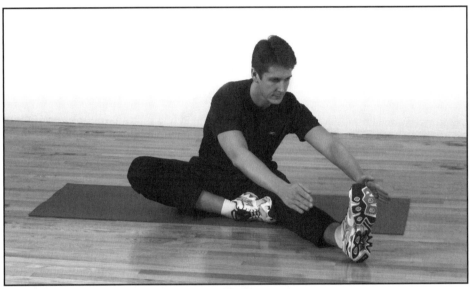

Step 2

Step 1. From your gluteal stretch, uncross and straighten your top leg out to your side.

Step 2. Exhale forcefully, tighten your abdominals, and reach toward your left foot to stretch your hamstrings and calves.

Step 3. Hold for 4 deep exhalations.

TARGET MUSCLES:
Biceps femoris (hamstrings), *gastrocnemius* and *soleus* (calf), and *adductors* (inner thighs).

TECHNIQUE TIPS:
Keep shoulders down while you reach; it's not how far you go, it's how you get there.

Stretch Series
Level 2

GOAL:

To stretch the inner thigh and leg muscles.

TARGET MUSCLES:

Biceps femoris (hamstring) and *adductors* (inner thighs).

TECHNIQUE TIPS:

Never force this stretch. Go down only as far as it's comfortable. Keep your *pelvic floor* and lower abdominal muscles tight as you stretch.

im
=X

122

ADDUCTOR STRETCH

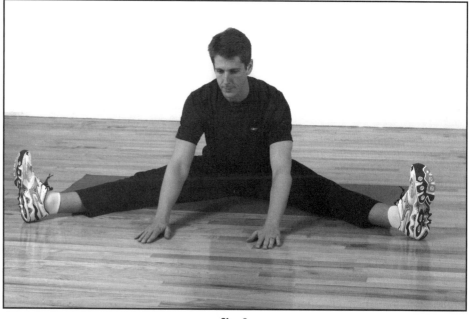

Step 2

Step 1. From your hamstring stretch, straighten your bent leg so that your legs form a wide V on the floor.

Step 2. Exhale forcefully, tighten your abdominals, lengthen your spine and reach forward to the center.

Step 3. Hold for 4 deep exhalations, keeping your legs as straight as possible.

Repeat the sequence on the left side.

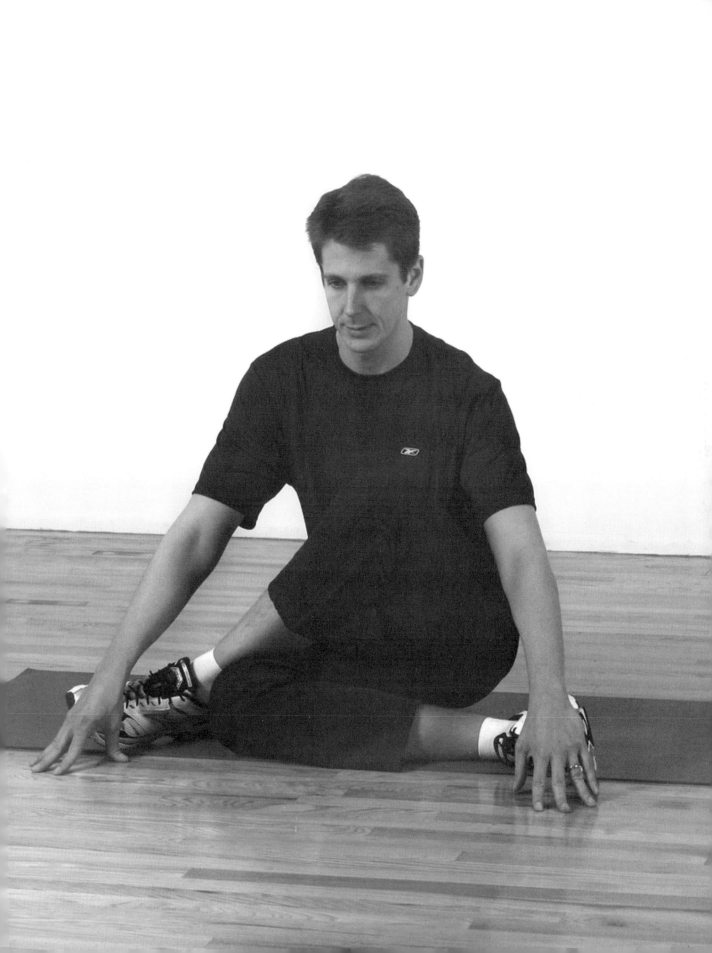

Chapter 14

Ab Series
Level 3

This sequence adds leg movement in addition to the abdominal and weight exercises of the previous ab series. Thus you are developing leg and hip flexibility while you are strengthening your trunk and shoulder muscles. It does require a bit of coordination so take your time learning these moves.

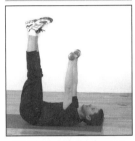

Exercise 1a

LEG EXTENSION & BENCH PRESS WITH HEAVY WEIGHTS OR ▸

Exercise 1b

LEG EXTENSION ABDOMINAL CURL & BENCH PRESS WITH HEAVY WEIGHTS

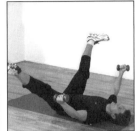

Exercise 2a

V STRETCH & PEC FLIES WITH LIGHT WEIGHTS OR ▸

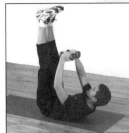

Exercise 2b

V STRETCH ABDOMINAL CURL & PEC FLIES WITH LIGHT WEIGHTS

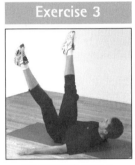

Exercise 3

ABDOMINAL CURL & DOUBLE LEG CIRCLE

GOAL:

Strengthen the abdominal and hip muscles while stretching the hamstrings.

TARGET MUSCLES:

Iliopsoas (hip flexors), *biceps femoris* (hamstrings), *latissimus dorsi* (upper back), *pectoralis* (chest), *biceps* and *triceps* (arms), and *deltoids* (shoulder) muscles.

TECHNIQUE TIPS:

Hold your shoulders down by engaging your back muscles.

$\dfrac{im}{=X}$

126

Exercise 1a

LEG EXTENSION & BENCH PRESS WITH HEAVY WEIGHTS

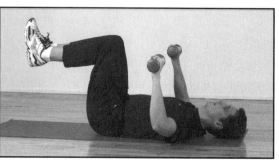

Step 1

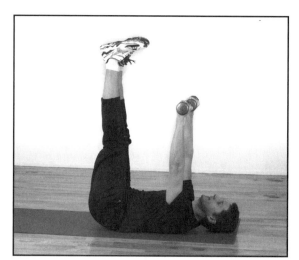

Step 2

OR

Step 1. Lie on your back with your knees bent into your chest. Take a weight in each hand. With your elbows out to the side and your forearms perpendicular to the floor, hold your weights up on either side of your chest, palms facing forward.

Step 2. Exhale forcefully, tighten your abdominals, and press the weights straight up while extending your legs straight up to a 90-degree angle.

Step 3. As you inhale, bend your arms and legs back to your starting position.

Step 4. Repeat 8 times slowly.

LEG EXTENSION ABDOMINAL CURL & BENCH PRESS WITH HEAVY WEIGHTS

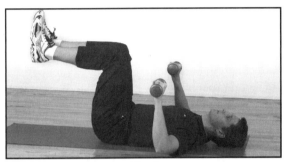

Step 1

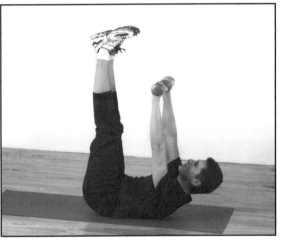

Step 2

This is the same exercise as #1a but with an ab curl.

Step 1. Lie on your back with your knees bent into your chest. Take a weight in each hand. With your elbows out to the side and your forearms perpendicular to the floor, hold your weights up on either side of your chest, palms facing forward.

Step 2. Exhale forcefully, tighten your abdominals, curl up, and press the weights straight up. At the same time, straighten your legs and extend them up at a 90-degree angle.

Step 3. As you inhale, lower yourself slowly back to your starting position.

Step 4. Repeat 8 times slowly.

GOAL:

Strengthen the abdominal, shoulder, and hip flexor muscles.

TARGET MUSCLES:

Same as the previous exercise plus the *transversus abdominis* (deepest abdominal layer).

TECHNIQUE TIPS:

Keep in mind that the weights are being used to increase your abdominal power more so than the shoulders, so don't worry if you don't feel fatigued in your shoulder muscles.

Ab Series
Level 3

GOAL:

Stabilize the spine and strengthen the upper body while increasing flexibility in the hip and legs.

TARGET MUSCLES:

Iliopsoas (hip flexors), *biceps femoris* (hamstrings), *adductors* (inner thighs), *latissimus dorsi* (upper back), *pectoralis* (chest), and *deltoids* (shoulder) muscles.

TECHNIQUE TIPS:

Keep your knees as straight as possible to increase the stretch.

V STRETCH & PEC FLIES WITH LIGHT WEIGHTS

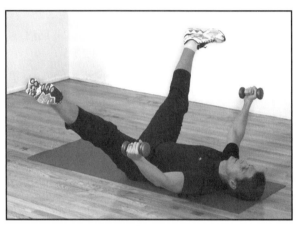

Step 2

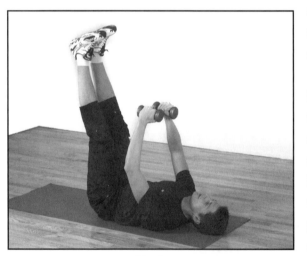

Step 3

Step 1. Still lying on your back with your knees bent into your chest, take a weight in each hand. Extend your arms and legs up to a 90-degree angle.

Step 2. Rotate your legs outward and open them to your sides; simultaneously reach your arms out to your sides with elbows slightly bent.

Step 3. Exhale forcefully, and raise your legs straight back up to a 90-degree angle with your inner thighs and heels touching (your toes point away from each other). At the same time, arc your arms up until they are directly over your chest, keeping your elbows slightly bent.

Step 4. As you inhale, bring your arms back to the open position so that they form a V. Exhale, and bring your legs together again while arcing your arms up.

Step 5. Repeat 8 times.

OR

V STRETCH ABDOMINAL CURL & PEC FLIES WITH LIGHT WEIGHTS

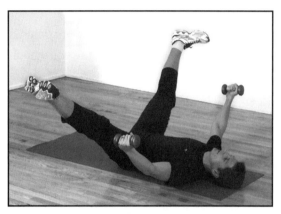

Step 2

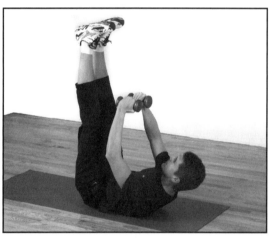

Step 3

This is the same exercise as #2a but with a curl.

Step 1. Still lying on your back with your knees bent into your chest, take a weight in each hand. Extend your arms and legs up to a 90-degree angle.

Step 2. Rotate your legs outward and open them to your sides; simultaneously reach your arms out to your sides with elbows slightly bent.

Step 3. Exhale forcefully, and raise your legs to a 90-degree angle with your inner thighs squeezing tight. At the same time, arc your arms up and curl.

Step 4. As you inhale, lower from the curl and open your arms and legs to stretch.

Step 5. Repeat 8 times.

GOAL:

Strengthen the abdominal wall while increasing hip range of motion.

TARGET MUSCLES:

Same as the previous exercise but plus the *transversus abdominis* (deepest abdominal layer), internal and *external oblique*s (intermediate abdominal layers), and *rectus abdominis* (superficial abdominal layer).

TECHNIQUE TIPS:

Use the forced exhalation breath to initiate this move; it will improve your core strength and hip flexibility.

Ab Series
Level 3

129

GOAL: Increase hip range of motion.

TARGET MUSCLES:

Transversus abdominis (deepest abdominal layer), *internal* and *external oblique*s (intermediate abdominal layers), *rectus abdominis* (superficial abdominal layer), *quadriceps* (thigh), *iliopsoas* (hip flexors), *biceps femoris* (hamstrings), and *adductors* (inner thighs).

TECHNIQUE TIPS:

Use the forced exhalation breath to pull the legs together and up to 90 degrees. You can try this with your knees slightly bent if that's easier. If you feel pain in your back, then STOP.

im=X

130

ABDOMINAL CURL & DOUBLE LEG CIRCLE

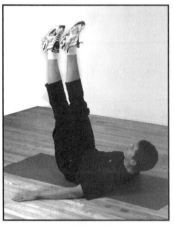

Step 1

Step 1. Still lying on your back with your knees bent into your chest, set the weights aside and place your hands on a low diagonal.

Step 2. Exhale forcefully, curl up until you feel your abdominals working, and lift both legs to about a 45-degree angle, keeping them rotated slightly outward.

Step 3. Make a circular movement with your legs. They should circle from a 90-degree angle and come back together at a 45-degree angle and up again. DO NOT LOWER FROM THE CURL.

Step 5. Repeat 8 times.

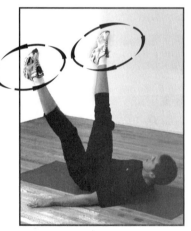

Step 2

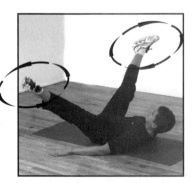

Step 3

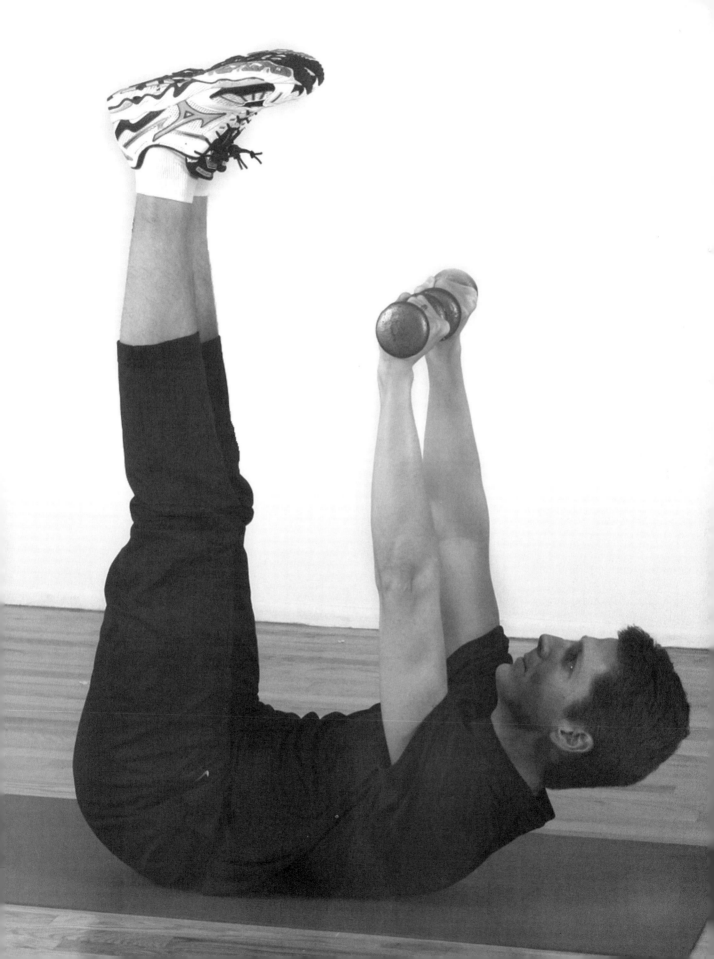

Back Series
Level 3

This series continues to target back and hip extensor muscles but adds an element of flexibility for your *quadriceps* and lower spine.

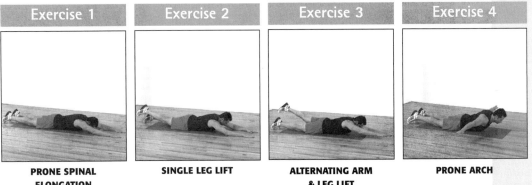

Exercise 1	Exercise 2	Exercise 3	Exercise 4
PRONE SPINAL ELONGATION	SINGLE LEG LIFT	ALTERNATING ARM & LEG LIFT	PRONE ARCH

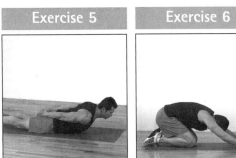

Exercise 5	Exercise 6
SHOULDER STRETCH	LOWER BACK STRETCH

GOAL:

Lengthen and decompress your spine.

TARGET MUSCLES:

Transversus abdominis (deepest abdominal layer), *internal* and *external obliques* (intermediate abdominal layers), *rectus abdominis* (superficial abdominal layer), *iliopsoas* (hip flexor), *erector spinae* (spine), *latissimus dorsi* (upper back), *levatores, rotatores, multifidus* (back), and *quadratus lumborum* (lower back) muscles.

TECHNIQUE TIPS:

Make sure that you feel the length through the hips and waist rather than lifting your shoulders to your ears.

PRONE SPINAL ELONGATION

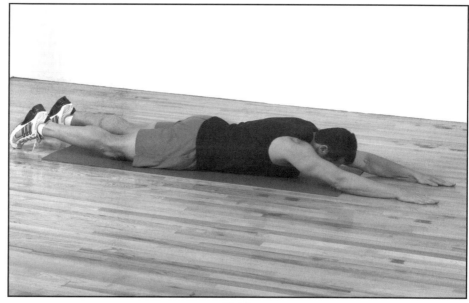

Step 1

Step 1. Lie on your stomach with your arms flat on the floor above your head and legs straight on the floor. Lengthen through the right arm and right leg by reaching them away from each other to stretch the right side of your waist and hips.

Step 2. Repeat with the left arm and left leg, stretching through the left side of your body.

Step 3. Then reach both arms and legs as long as you can. Imagine that there is more space between each vertebra and maintain this extended spine through your workout.

Exercise 2

SINGLE LEG LIFT

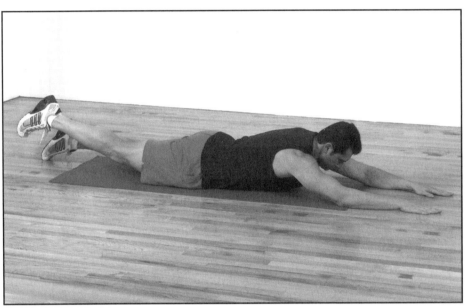

Step 2

Step 1. Still lying on your stomach with your arms flat on the floor above your head and your legs straight, press your forearms into the floor. Anchor your pelvis by tightening your hip and lower abdominal muscles, and look down to keep your neck relaxed.

Step 2. Exhale forcefully, reach the right leg long out of the hip, and lift it up slightly.

Step 3. Inhale as you lower your leg slowly to your starting position.

Step 4. Repeat 15 times, then switch sides.

GOAL:
Strengthen the hip extensors while stabilizing the spine.

TARGET MUSCLES:
Transversus abdominis (deepest abdominal layer), *erector spinae* (spine), *multifidus* (back), *quadratus lumborum* (lower back), *biceps femoris* (hamstrings), *gluteal* (butt), and *pelvic floor* muscles.

TECHNIQUE TIPS:
Keep your spine as still as possible.

Back Series
Level 3

135

GOAL:

Strengthen the back muscles and increase spinal and hip length.

TARGET MUSCLES:

Transversus abdominis (deepest abdominal layer), *erector spinae* (spine), *multifidus* (back), *quadratus lumborum* (lower back), *biceps femoris* (hamstrings), *gluteal* (butt), *pelvic floor*, *latissimus dorsi, trapezius* (upper back), *deltoids* (shoulder), *levator scapula*, and *rhomboids* (shoulder) muscles.

TECHNIQUE TIPS:

Keep your shoulders down while reaching overhead. Lengthen your spine by stretching your arm and leg.

136

ALTERNATING ARM & LEG LIFT

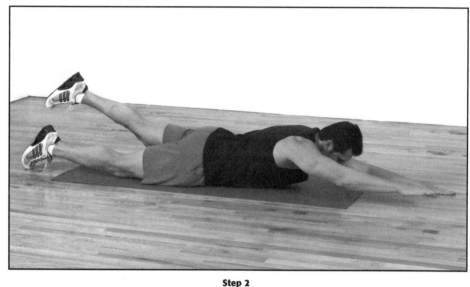

Step 2

Step 1. Still lying on your stomach with your arms flat on the floor above your head and your legs straight, press your forearms into the floor. Anchor your pelvis by tightening your hip and lower abdominal muscles, and look down to keep your neck relaxed.

Step 2. Exhale forcefully, tighten your abdominals, and lift your right arm and left leg slightly.

Step 3. Inhale as you lower your arm and leg back to your starting position.

Step 4. Repeat 10 times on each side.

Exercise 4

PRONE ARCH

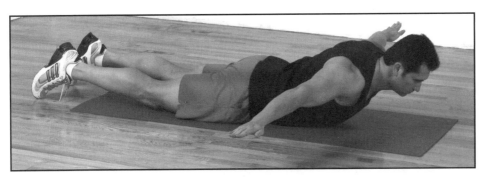

Step 1

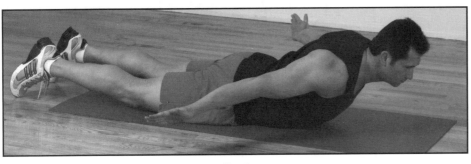

Step 2

Step 1. Still lying on your stomach with your legs straight, reach your arms out to the side. Lengthen your legs and press them into the mat.

Step 2. Exhale forcefully, tighten your abdominals, arch your upper back, and reach your arms back toward your hips.

Step 3. Inhale as you lower yourself back to your starting position.

Step 4. Repeat 10 times.

TARGET MUSCLES:

Transversus abdominis (deepest abdominal layer), *erector spinae* (spine), *latissimus dorsi* (upper back), *multifidus* (back), *quadratus lumborum* (lower back), *triceps* (arms), *deltoids* (shoulder), *trapezius* (upper back), *biceps femoris* (hamstrings), *gluteal* (butt), and *pelvic floor* muscles.

TECHNIQUE TIPS:

Focus on contracting your lower abs and *pelvic floor* to anchor your hips as you lift up. Keep the abdominals engaged throughout the exercise.

Back Series
Level 3

GOAL:

Increase flexibility at the shoulder joint while strengthening the back.

TARGET MUSCLES:

Transversus abdominis (deepest abdominal layer), *erector spinae* (spine), *latissimus dorsi* (upper back), *multifidus* (back), *quadratus lumborum* (lower back), *levator scapula, rhomboids, serratus anterior, deltoids* (shoulder), and other shoulder muscles.

TECHNIQUE TIPS:

Keep the neck muscles relaxed and abdominals tight.

im
=X

138

Exercise 5

SHOULDER STRETCH

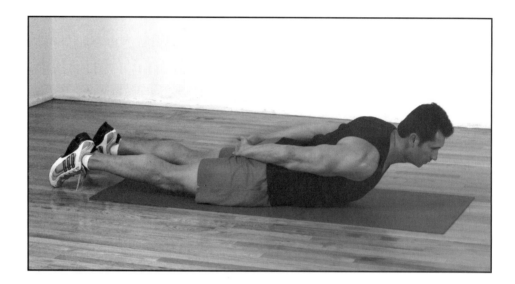

Step 2

Step 1. Still lying on your stomach with your legs straight, clasp your hands behind you.

Step 2. Exhale forcefully, tighten your abdominals, extend your arms, and arch your upper back.

Step 3. Hold for 4 deep exhalations.

Exercise 6

LOWER BACK STRETCH

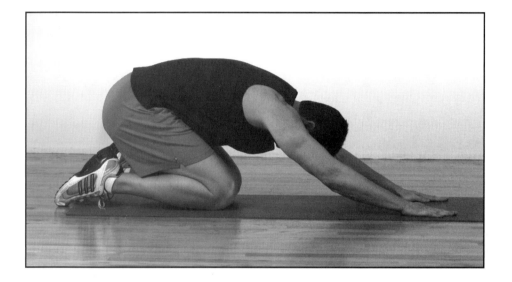

Step 1

Step 1. Sit back on your heels, or as far as you can, reaching your arms overhead.

Step 2. Breathe deeply into the spine and hip area to relax the muscles you have just worked.

YOU HAVE NOW COMPLETED THE *Pilates for Men* WORKOUT!

GOAL:
Stretch the lower back and hip muscles.

TARGET MUSCLES:
Erector spinae (spine), *quadratus lumborum* (lower back), and *multifidus* (back).

TECHNIQUE TIPS:
If you feel any pain in the knees, do not do this stretch.

Back Series
Level 3

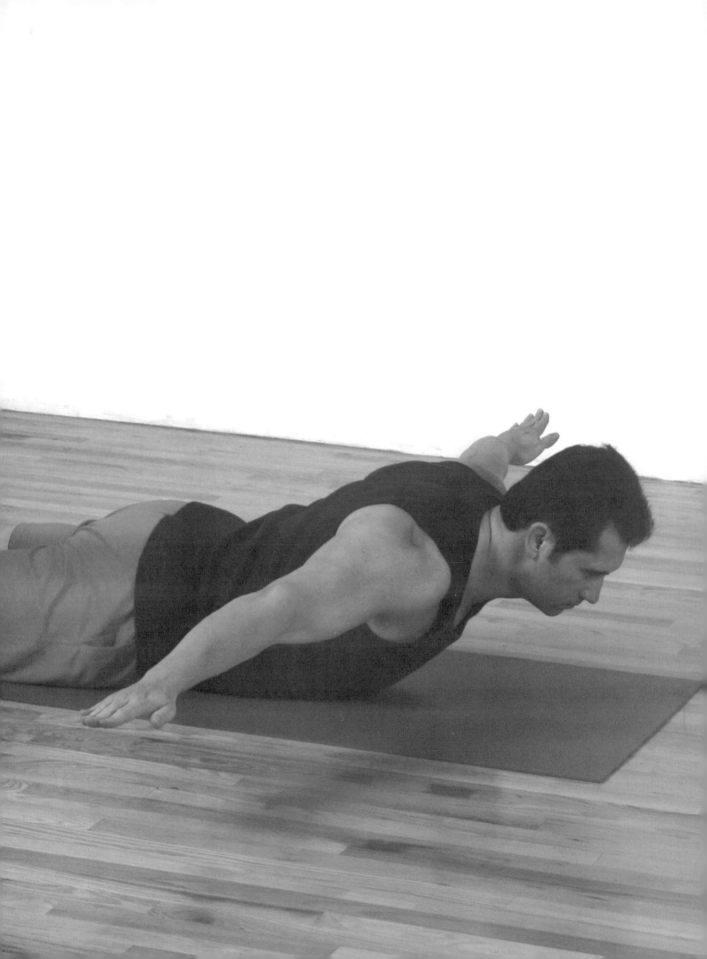

Chapter
16

Maintain Your Motivation

Congratulations! You have taken the first step to improving your health and strengthening your body. IM=X Pilates floor exercise routines are incredibly challenging for anyone, no matter your fitness experience. Maintaining a level of enthusiasm long-term is even harder. Motivation can be difficult because there are multiple factors that influence our ability to commit to fitness—work, family, available time, stress, etc.

Methods of getting and staying motivated vary from person to person. I have long been a believer of "something is better than nothing" and "more is better." In fact, the Surgeon General of the U.S. recommends no less than 30 minutes of exercise a day. We have members at our Madison Avenue Studio who show up five times a week to take the floor and machine-based Upper Body, Interval Training, Cardio, Stretch, Lower Body classes. We also have members who join and show up one time per week for their favorite class. Each person has his or her own needs and goals, and simply committing to any exercise program is a great first step.

Pilates can be a successful path for reaching your fitness goals. Goals for exercising can be broad, and different types of people reap the benefits of exercise for different reasons. Some are athletes whose job is dependent upon solid exercise programs and injury prevention; others are seniors who need fitness to stay healthy and active; still others are using Pilates to relieve back pain. Some simply want to fit into their jeans. One universal truth is that it is easier to stay motivated when you see the results of your hard work.

But if you are looking for a reason to exercise, focus on the health benefits. Regular exercise helps stave off a variety of health problems—diabetes, obesity, heart disease, cancer, to name a few. It truly is the elixir to youth and helps you live a better life. Exercise helps you look and feel good. According to the medical community, exercise is proclaimed to be an inexpensive and effective drug to help depression or anxiety. I call it the stress buster!

Regular exercise builds strength and will positively affect activities that you do every day. For overweight and inactive individuals, even simple movements can become challenging (i.e. walking, bending, sex). Becoming active is the key to improving body composition and stimulating weight loss. Strength-building of any kind (i.e. IM=X Pilates, weight lifting, cycling) increases muscles mass. Muscle tissue is more metabolically active than fat tissue and thus yields more calorie building.

Body composition changes occur after the age of 30. In fact, aging is characterized by muscle wasting (sarcopenia) unless resistance or weight training is used to offset the process. A well-rounded fitness program of muscle building and cardiovascular activity allows overweight individuals to be a little more liberal with their food consumption while maintaining a favorable ratio of muscle to fat. In other words, weight loss can occur by exercise alone even though it usually is done in combination with dieting.

The mounds of data on the morbidity and mortality associated with not exercising should be enough to get you moving. By participating in regular exercise you will limit your weight gain and protect yourself from a host of unwanted diseases.

If you are motivated by well-being…
If you are motivated by accomplishment…
If you are motivated to have more muscle endurance for sex…
If you are motivated to lower your high blood pressure…
If you are motivated to make sure you are around for your family…
If you are motivated to fit into those jeans…
If you are motivated to be the strongest you can be…
If you are motivated to improve your game…

Then, just keep exercising and use IM=X Pilates for your core strength.

The *Pilates for Men* Program

As described in Chapter 2, the twelve series of movements in this book are designed to build upon each other. You should always begin with the Foundational Series, which includes exercises to reinforce the five fundamental IM=X principles: spinal elongation, forced exhalation, pelvic, ribcage, and spine stabilization. These five principles should be applied to every movement, so never skip them! You will get the most of your workout if you follow each series exactly. If you find any single exercise (other than the five fundamental exercises) too difficult or painful, first try to modify it according to the instructions. If it's still a problem, then skip it and move on to the next exercise.

No warm-up, cool-down, or stretching routines are necessary, since those are all built in to the workouts presented here. Your *Pilates for Men* routine can serve as a warm-up to your regular gym routine, or you can do it on separate days if that is more convenient.

For the first two weeks, perform all of the exercises without weights. Then, when you feel comfortable with the techniques, add light weights as indicated. The Level 1 Workout should take about half an hour to complete. Do this workout three days a week.

Foundational Series (Ab Series Level 1)

1) Roll Down
2) Double Knee Stretch
3) Spinal Elongation
4) Forced Exhalation
5) Pelvic Stabilization with ring
6a) Abdominal Curls with ring **OR**
6b) Abdominal Curls with ring and light weights
7a) Oblique Curls with ring **OR**
7b) Oblique Curls with ring and light weights
8) Lower Back Mobilization with ring
9) Abdominal Curl & Bench Press with ring and heavy weights
10) Oblique Curl & Bench Press with ring and heavy weights
11a) Reverse Curl with ring **OR**
11b) Reverse Curl & Bench Press with ring and heavy weights

Stretch Series Level 1

1) Knee Side/External Rotation/Knee Side
2) Knee Stretch
3) Hamstring Stretch with ring
4) Bent Leg Knee Extension with ring
5) Straight Leg Knee Extension with ring
6) Lower Back & Hamstring Stretch with ring

Back Series Level 1

1) Arch
2) Push-Up Hold
3) Inverted V Hold
4) Leg Lift in a Push-Up Hold
5) Cat Back Stretch

The *Pilates for Men* Program

Ab & Hip Series Level 1

1) Bent Knee Abdominal Curl

2a) Bent Knee Abdominal Curl & Bench Press with heavy weights **OR**

2b) Extended Knee Abdominal Curl & Bench Press with heavy weights

3) Cross Knee Stretch

4) Extended Leg Abdominal Curl

5a) Extended Leg Abdominal Curl & Bench Press with heavy weights **OR**

5b) Leg Lift Abdominal Curl & Bench Press with heavy weights

6) Overhead Stretch

In Weeks 5-8, you will be adding the Level 2 series to the Level 1 workout for a longer and more intense routine. You should do the full routine, which should take about an hour, at least once a week. On the other two days, you can use the shorter Level 2 Alternate routine, which takes only about half an hour. For the first two weeks, you should stick to the lighter weights. Then, when you feel comfortable with the movements, you can move up to the heavier weights.

Foundational Series (Ab Series Level 1)

1) Roll Down
2) Double Knee Stretch
3) Spinal Elongation
4) Forced Exhalation
5) Pelvic Stabilization with ring
6a) Abdominal Curls with ring **OR**
6b) Abdominal Curls with ring and light weights
7a) Oblique Curls with ring **OR**
7b) Oblique Curls with ring and light weights
8) Lower Back Mobilization with ring
9) Abdominal Curl & Bench Press with ring and heavy weights
10) Oblique Curl & Bench Press with ring and heavy weights
11a) Reverse Curl with ring **OR**
11b) Reverse Curl & Bench Press with ring and heavy weights

Stretch Series Level 1

1) Knee Side/External Rotation/Knee Side
2) Knee Stretch
3) Hamstring Stretch with ring
4) Bent Leg Knee Extension with ring
5) Straight Leg Knee Extension with ring
6) Lower Back & Hamstring Stretch with ring

The *Pilates for Men* Program

Ab Series Level 2

1) Core Recruitment with ring
2a) Extended Leg Abdominal Curls with ring **OR**
2b) Extended Leg Abdominal Curls with ring and light weights
3a) Extended Leg Oblique Curls with ring **OR**
3b) Extended Leg Oblique Curls with ring and light weights
4) Lower Back & Hamstring Stretch with ring
5) Abdominal Curl & Pec Flies with ring and light weights
6) Oblique Curl & Pec Flies with ring and light weights
7) Extended Leg Reverse Curl & Bench Press with ring and heavy weights
8) Extended Leg Reverse Curl & Pec Flies with ring and heavy weights

Back Series Level 1

1) Arch
2) Push-Up Hold
3) Inverted V Hold
4) Leg Lift in a Push-Up Hold
5) Cat Back Stretch

Ab & Hip Series Level 1

1) Bent Knee Abdominal Curl
2a) Bent Knee Abdominal Curl & Bench Press with heavy weights **OR**
2b) Extended Knee Abdominal Curl & Bench Press with heavy weights
3) Cross Knee Stretch
4) Extended Leg Abdominal Curl
5a) Extended Leg Abdominal Curl & Bench Press with heavy weights **OR**
5b) Leg Lift Abdominal Curl & Bench Press with heavy weights
6) Overhead Stretch

Back Series Level 2

1) Arch
2) Push-Ups
3) Inverted V Push-Ups
4) Leg Lift with Push-Ups

Ab & Hip Series Level 2

1a) Abdominal Curl Knee Changes **OR**

1b) Abdominal Curl Leg Changes

2a) Abdominal Curl Knee Changes & Pec Flies with light weights **OR**

2b) Abdominal Curl Leg Changes & Pec Flies with light weights

3a) Abdominal Curl Knee Changes & Bench Press with heavy weights
OR

3b) Abdominal Curl Leg Changes & Bench Press with heavy weights

4a) Oblique Curl Knee Changes **OR**

4b) Oblique Curl Leg Changes

Stretch Series Level 2

1) Back Extension Hold

2) Hip Stretch

3) Gluteal Stretch

4) Hamstring Stretch

5) Adductor Stretch

LEVEL 2 ALTERNATE
Foundational Series (Ab Series Level 1)

1) Roll Down
2) Double Knee Stretch
3) Spinal Elongation
4) Forced Exhalation
5) Pelvic Stabilization with ring
6a) Abdominal Curls with ring **OR**
6b) Abdominal Curls with ring and light weights
7a) Oblique Curls with ring **OR**
7b) Oblique Curls with ring and light weights
8) Lower Back Mobilization with ring
9) Abdominal Curl & Bench Press with ring and heavy weights
10) Oblique Curl & Bench Press with ring and heavy weights
11a) Reverse Curl with ring **OR**
11b) Reverse Curl & Bench Press with ring and heavy weights

Ab Series Level 2

1) Core Recruitment with ring
2a) Extended Leg Abdominal Curls with ring **OR**
2b) Extended Leg Abdominal Curls with ring and light weights
3a) Extended Leg Oblique Curls with ring **OR**
3b) Extended Leg Oblique Curls with ring and light weights
4) Lower Back & Hamstring Stretch with ring
5) Abdominal Curl & Pec Flies with ring and light weights
6) Oblique Curl & Pec Flies with ring and light weights
7) Extended Leg Reverse Curl & Bench Press with ring and heavy weights
8) Extended Leg Reverse Curl & Pec Flies with ring and heavy weights

Back Series Level 1

1) Arch
2) Push-Up Hold
3) Inverted V Hold
4) Leg Lift in a Push-Up Hold
5) Cat Back Stretch

Back Series Level 2

1) Arch
2) Push-Ups
3) Inverted V Push-Ups
4) Leg Lift with Push-Ups

Ab & Hip Series Level 2

1a) Abdominal Curl Knee Changes **OR**
1b) Abdominal Curl Leg Changes
2a) Abdominal Curl Knee Changes & Pec Flies with light weights **OR**
2b) Abdominal Curl Leg Changes & Pec Flies with light weights
3a) Abdominal Curl Knee Changes & Bench Press with heavy weights **OR**
3b) Abdominal Curl Leg Changes & Bench Press with heavy weights
4a) Oblique Curl Knee Changes **OR**
4b) Oblique Curl Leg Changes

Stretch Series Level 2

1) Back Extension Hold
2) Hip Stretch
3) Gluteal Stretch
4) Hamstring Stretch
5) Adductor Stretch

In Weeks 9–12, add the Level 3 and Special Series to the Level 2 Alternate workout for a super-intense hour-long routine once a week. On the other two days, use the Level 3 Alternate half-hour routine.

Foundational Series (Ab Series Level 1)

1) Roll Down
2) Double Knee Stretch
3) Spinal Elongation
4) Forced Exhalation
5) Pelvic Stabilization with ring
6a) Abdominal Curls with ring **OR**
6b) Abdominal Curls with ring and light weights
7a) Oblique Curls with ring **OR**
7b) Oblique Curls with ring and light weights
8) Lower Back Mobilization with ring
9) Abdominal Curl & Bench Press with ring and heavy weights
10) Oblique Curl & Bench Press with ring and heavy weights
11a) Reverse Curl with ring **OR**
11b) Reverse Curl & Bench Press with ring and heavy weights

Ab Series Level 2

1) Core Recruitment with ring
2a) Extended Leg Abdominal Curls with ring **OR**
2b) Extended Leg Abdominal Curls with ring and light weights
3a) Extended Leg Oblique Curls with ring **OR**
3b) Extended Leg Oblique Curls with ring and light weights
4) Lower Back & Hamstring Stretch with ring
5) Abdominal Curl & Pec Flies with ring and light weights
6) Oblique Curl & Pec Flies with ring and light weights
7) Extended Leg Reverse Curl & Bench Press with ring and heavy weights
8) Extended Leg Reverse Curl & Pec Flies with ring and heavy weights

Back Series Level 2

1) Arch
2) Push-Ups
3) Inverted V Push-Ups
4) Leg Lift with Push-Ups

Ab & Hip Series Level 2

1a) Abdominal Curl Knee Changes **OR**
1b) Abdominal Curl Leg Changes
2a) Abdominal Curl Knee Changes & Pec Flies with light weights **OR**
2b) Abdominal Curl Leg Changes & Pec Flies with light weights
3a) Abdominal Curl Knee Changes & Bench Press with heavy weights **OR**
3b) Abdominal Curl Leg Changes & Bench Press with heavy weights
4a) Oblique Curl Knee Changes **OR**
4b) Oblique Curl Leg Changes

Lateral Moves

1) Lateral Stretch
2) Lateral Push-Up
3) Single Leg Circle
4) Single Leg Lift
5) Double Leg Lift

Spine Stabilizer Series

1) Seated Core Recruitment with ring
2) Spine Curl with ring
3) Spine Rotation with ring
4) Spine Reach with ring
5) Spine Curl & Bench Press with heavy weights

Stretch Series Level 2

1) Back Extension Hold
2) Hip Stretch
3) Gluteal Stretch
4) Hamstring Stretch
5) Adductor Stretch

Ab Series Level 3

1a) Leg Extension & Bench Press **OR**
1b) Leg Extension Abdominal Curl & Bench Press with heavy weights
2a) V Stretch & Pec Flies with light weights **OR**
2b) V Stretch Abdominal Curl & Pec Flies with light weights
3) Abdominal Curl & Double Leg Circle

Back Series Level 3

1) Prone Spinal Elongation
2) Single Leg Lift
3) Alternating Arm & Leg Lift
4) Prone Arch
5) Shoulder Stretch
6) Lower Back Stretch

LEVEL 3 ALTERNATE
Foundational Series (Ab Series Level 1)

1) Roll Down
2) Double Knee Stretch
3) Spinal Elongation
4) Forced Exhalation
5) Pelvic Stabilization with ring
6a) Abdominal Curls with ring **OR**
6b) Abdominal Curls with ring and light weights
7a) Oblique Curls with ring **OR**
7b) Oblique Curls with ring and light weights
8) Lower Back Mobilization with ring
9) Abdominal Curl & Bench Press with ring and heavy weights
10) Oblique Curl & Bench Press with ring and heavy weights
11a) Reverse Curl with ring **OR**
11b) Reverse Curl & Bench Press with ring and heavy weights

Lateral Moves

1) Lateral Stretch
2) Lateral Push-Up
3) Single Leg Circle
4) Single Leg Lift
5) Double Leg Lift

Spine Stabilizer Series

1) Seated Core Recruitment with ring
2) Spine Curl with ring
3) Spine Rotation with ring
4) Spine Reach with ring
5) Spine Curl & Bench Press with heavy weights

The *Pilates for Men* Program

Ab Series Level 3

1a) Leg Extension & Bench Press **OR**
1b) Leg Extension Abdominal Curl & Bench Press with heavy weights
2a) V Stretch & Pec Flies with light weights **OR**
2b) V Stretch Abdominal Curl & Pec Flies with light weights
3) Abdominal Curl & Double Leg Circle

Back Series Level 3

1) Prone Spinal Elongation
2) Single Leg Lift
3) Alternating Arm & Leg Lift
4) Prone Arch
5) Shoulder Stretch
6) Lower Back Stretch

After you have completed Week 12, you have several options. If you are still having problems with any of the exercises, continue to work with the modifications until you have mastered the original exercises. You may want to drop down to the Level 1 or Level 2 routine to give your muscles a break.

If you feel comfortable with the Level 3 routine, but aren't ready to move on to anything more intense, you can maintain your three-day-a-week routine and slowly add weights. Also, every two weeks or so, extend your program to include all of the series in this book for a 90-minute super-strong workout:

Foundational Series (Ab Series Level 1)

1) Roll Down
2) Double Knee Stretch
3) Spinal Elongation
4) Forced Exhalation
5) Pelvic Stabilization with ring
6a) Abdominal Curls with ring **OR**
6b) Abdominal Curls with ring and light weights
7a) Oblique Curls with ring **OR**
7b) Oblique Curls with ring and light weights
8) Lower Back Mobilization with ring
9) Abdominal Curl & Bench Press with ring and heavy weights
10) Oblique Curl & Bench Press with ring and heavy weights
11a) Reverse Curl with ring **OR**
11b) Reverse Curl & Bench Press with ring and heavy weights

Stretch Series Level 1

1) Knee Side/External Rotation/Knee Side
2) Knee Stretch
3) Hamstring Stretch with ring
4) Bent Leg Knee Extension with ring
5) Straight Leg Knee Extension with ring
6) Lower Back & Hamstring Stretch with ring

The *Pilates for Men* Program

Ab Series Level 2

1) Core Recruitment with ring
2a) Extended Leg Abdominal Curls with ring **OR**
2b) Extended Leg Abdominal Curls with ring and light weights
3a) Extended Leg Oblique Curls with ring **OR**
3b) Extended Leg Oblique Curls with ring and light weights
4) Lower Back & Hamstring Stretch with ring
5) Abdominal Curl & Pec Flies with ring and light weights
6) Oblique Curl & Pec Flies with ring and light weights
7) Extended Leg Reverse Curl & Bench Press with ring and heavy weights
8) Extended Leg Reverse Curl & Pec Flies with ring and heavy weights

Back Series Level 1

1) Arch
2) Push-Up Hold
3) Inverted V Hold
4) Leg Lift in a Push-Up Hold
5) Cat Back Stretch

Ab & Hip Series Level 1

1) Bent Knee Abdominal Curl
2a) Bent Knee Abdominal Curl & Bench Press with heavy weights **OR**
2b) Extended Knee Abdominal Curl & Bench Press with heavy weights
3) Cross Knee Stretch
4) Extended Leg Abdominal Curl
5a) Extended Leg Abdominal Curl & Bench Press with heavy weights **OR**
5b) Leg Lift Abdominal Curl & Bench Press with heavy weights
6) Overhead Stretch

Back Series Level 2

1) Arch
2) Push-Ups
3) Inverted V Push-Ups
4) Leg Lift with Push-Ups

Ab & Hip Series Level 2

1a) Abdominal Curl Knee Changes **OR**

1b) Abdominal Curl Leg Changes

2a) Abdominal Curl Knee Changes & Pec Flies with light weights **OR**

2b) Abdominal Curl Leg Changes & Pec Flies with light weights

3a) Abdominal Curl Knee Changes & Bench Press with heavy weights **OR**

3b) Abdominal Curl Leg Changes & Bench Press with heavy weights

4a) Oblique Curl Knee Changes **OR**

4b) Oblique Curl Leg Changes

Lateral Moves

1) Lateral Stretch

2) Lateral Push-Up

3) Single Leg Circle

4) Single Leg Lift

5) Double Leg Lift

Spine Stabilizer Series

1) Seated Core Recruitment with ring

2) Spine Curl with ring

3) Spine Rotation with ring

4) Spine Reach with ring

5) Spine Curl & Bench Press with heavy weights

Stretch Series Level 2

1) Back Extension Hold

2) Hip Stretch

3) Gluteal Stretch

4) Hamstring Stretch

5) Adductor Stretch

Ab Series Level 3

1a) Leg Extension & Bench Press **OR**

1b) Leg Extension Abdominal Curl & Bench Press with heavy weights

2a) V Stretch & Pec Flies with light weights **OR**

2b) V Stretch Abdominal Curl & Pec Flies with light weights

3) Abdominal Curl & Double Leg Circle

The *Pilates for Men* Program

Back Series Level 3

1) Prone Spinal Elongation
2) Single Leg Lift
3) Alternating Arm & Leg Lift
4) Prone Arch
5) Shoulder Stretch
6) Lower Back Stretch

If you have mastered all of the techniques, and are still looking for something stronger, you are ready for the Xerciser (the improved IM=X version of Joseph Pilates's Reformer machine). See Appendix II for more information.

Making It More Challenging

Congratulations! You've made it through a tough workout—hopefully many times! —and are now feeling the effects that the *Pilates for Men* program can have on your body in just a short period of time. Your body is toned, your core is stronger, and your spine, hips, legs and shoulders are more flexible. So what is next? Can you go farther with this type of exercise? Yes!

There are several options for you to expand on the program you've just mastered and keep the excitement going:

    1) vary your floor routine with the IM=X Pilates Video Series

        2) take a session on the Xercizer

            3) get an Xercizer for home use

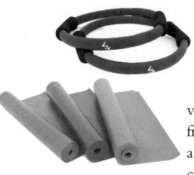

You can vary and expand your floor routines by working with the **IM=X Pilates Video Series**. The routines in the videos are complementary yet different from those in *Pilates for Men*. You will need a mat, ring and weighted body bar (which can be ordered at www.imxpilates.com or 800.IMX.1336). We have five workouts, ranging from 30 minutes to one hour that will keep you challenged and will, with regular practice, build upon the great techniques that you have learned in this book.

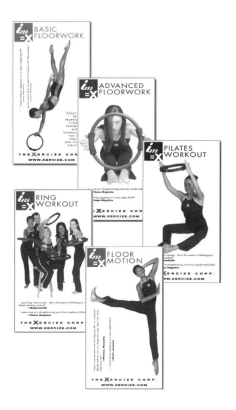

- **Basic Floorwork:** A challenging program which familiarizes you with IM=X Pilates moves and builds up core strength (45 minutes)

- **Advanced Floorwork:** Offers increased speed and intensity, plus the added challenge of a weighted body bar—it will push your body to the limit (40 minutes)

- **Pilates Floorwork:** Incorporates new exercises from traditional pilates for a longer workout routine. (60 minutes)

- **Ring Workout:** A quick but intense abdominal workout that tests your coordination and core muscle endurance (30 minutes)

- **Floor Motion:** Creative and complex choreography requires abdominal strength and control and focuses on fluid movement to increase flexibility.
(35 minutes)

The most ideal plan for taking IM=X Pilates to the next level is to find a studio near you and take private or semi-private sessions from a certified instructor. **The IM=X Pilates Studio** is a franchised business, with our headquarters and flagship located in New York City. The franchised studio network offers advanced training in both IM=X Pilates Floor and Reformer (our patented version is called the Xercizer) programs.

The Xercizer allows you to develop strength and flexibility in all muscles and joints using spring resistance, pulleys, a sliding carriage, jump platform, lumbar support and a wide range of workouts. Many of the

Making It More
Challenging

moves on the Xercizer develop functional strength through a full range of motion which is beneficial for overall posture and spine health as well as sports performance.

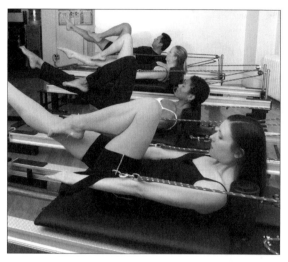

The studio network offers you a choice of many different workouts. You can experience specialized routines for golf and tennis, or build strength in specific areas with Lower Body, Upper Body, Back Strength, and Interval Training formats. You even have the option of adding heart rate training into your Pilates routine with the Cardio Xercizer workouts.

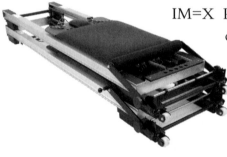

IM=X Pilates Studios are opening around the country, making it easier for more people to experience this unique fitness program. There is an efficiency to strength and flexibility training on the Xercizer because there are no breaks or lengthy equipment adjustments as can occur with traditional weight machines; thus, you accomplish more in less time. You will definitely find that the Xercizer brings a new level of challenge to your body.

If an IM=X Pilates Studio is not available near you, you may be able to find a gym with a certified IM=X Pilates trainer. We have been certifying instructors for over 8 years at our certification centers in New York and California. In summary, having a couple of sessions with a qualified teacher will help you perfect your technique, intensify trunk stabilization and improve your workout so that you grow stronger.

Glossary

ABDOMINAL WALL

The abdominal wall consists of four abdominal muscles: *rectus abdominis*, *internal oblique*, *external oblique* and *transversus abdominis*.

The *transversus abdominis* is the deepest supportive layer. The *transversus abdominis* contracts with the *pelvic floor* to stabilize the torso. Exterior to the *transversus abdominis* is the *internal oblique*. The *external oblique* lies near the lower eight ribs. The *transversus abdominis*, *internal oblique*, and *external oblique* have been shown to contract with the use of a forced exhalation. The *rectus abdominis* is the most superficial.

ADAPTIVE SHORTENING

Decreases in flexibility, spinal length, and mobility due to poor posture and/or repetitive stress.

BIOMECHANICS

The analysis of the postures and muscle synergy patterns that facilitate stabilization and exercise. Biomechanics is a tool for examining muscle activity in motion as it contributes to movement.

CONCENTRIC CONTRACTION

A shortening of the muscle as it exerts more force than the outside resistance.

CORE MUSCLE STRENGTH

A core set of muscles which support the integrity of the spine and hips including the four abdominal muscles, hip flexors, extensors, *pelvic floor,* and spinal muscles (particularly the intermediate and deepest layers of back muscles).

DECONDITIONING

Results from inactivity and includes a decrease in cardiovascular, neuro-muscular, and metabolic function.

DYSFUNCTION

A loss of function and mobility due to adaptive shortening of soft tissue and muscle.

END FEEL

The point at which the end of a stretch is reached. It is good to sense where your end feel is so that you do not overstretch.

FLAT LOWER BACK POSTURE

A posture characterized by a decreased lumbar curve with posterior tilting of the pelvis. This body position is often accompanied by tight hip muscles and chronic lower back pain.

FORCED EXHALATION

A technique of exhalation in which resistance is given to the outflow of air in order to facilitate a stronger contraction of the *transversus abdominis, internal oblique, external oblique, pelvic floor* and *diaphragm* muscles.

FORWARD HEAD POSTURE

Characterized by an increased forward position of the cervical and upper thoracic vertebrae. Often results in neck tension and pain.

IDEOKINETIC FACILITATION

Refers to the verbal cues of imagery which are used repeatedly to facilitate proper posture in exercise. Research has shown that imagined activity results in a 10% muscle response. Imagery is preferred to static commands for postural change because it encourages sensory feedback and muscle efficiency. For example: The instruction to "float the head" prior to a lifting a weight overhead helps to keep the exercise in the appropriate muscle groups not in the neck.

ISOMETRIC CONTRACTION
A static contraction as used in stabilization exercise. In general, the stabilization techniques use isometric contractions of many trunk muscles.

KYPHOSIS
A posture characterized by increased thoracic curve, rounded shoulders, and a forward head position. Corrected with a combination of manual traction, muscle setting, and stabilization exercises.

LENGTH-TENSION RELATIONSHIP
The optimum length at which a muscle can exert maximum force is slightly greater than the resting length of the muscle. True for all types of contraction. This is a key reason for increasing muscle and joint length at the spine and limbs during resistance training.

MOVEMENT EFFICIENCY
Minimal effort coupled with muscle synergy precision creates superior coordination and efficiency (i.e. a baseball pitcher trains to facilitate ease in the hips, spine, and shoulder as he throws).

MUSCLE SYNERGY
A muscle synergy is a contraction of key muscles and an inhibition of others to create more power and endurance in movement. Also thought of as distinct from single-muscle strength training as a more functional approach to muscle building for sports.

NEUTRAL SPINE POSITION
The natural alignment of the spine without flattening the cervical, thoracic, or lumbar curves. In the IM=X program the client is instructed to find a neutral spine and then lengthen slightly beyond it to prevent com-

Glossary

pression of the spinal segments during abdominal or back strengthening (also known as Spinal Elongation).

POSTURAL DYSFUNCTION
Poor posture characterized by adaptive shortening of the soft tissues and muscles of the back often leading to disc degeneration and height loss.

SPECIFICITY OF TRAINING
Take into consideration the precursors to injury by strengthening the postural and core muscles for injury prevention. Program design for athletes concentrates on improving the movement process for specific skills or countering repetitive motion by strengthening the weaker non–dominant movement patterns.